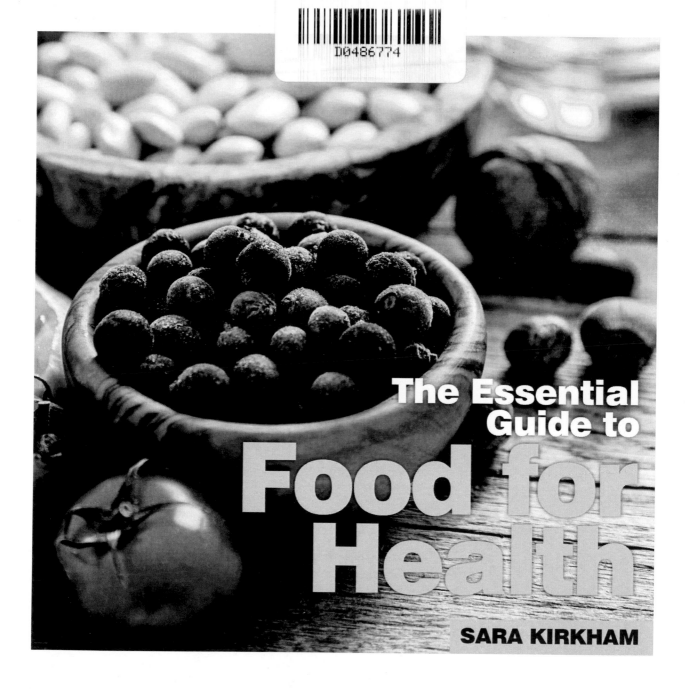

The Essential Guide to
Food for Health

SARA KIRKHAM

Published in Great Britain in 2018 by
need2know
Remus House
Coltsfoot Drive
Peterborough
PE2 9BF
Telephone 01733 898103
www.need2knowbooks.co.uk

Contents

Introduction

What could be better than finding an easy, inexpensive and healthy way to make you feel and look the picture of health? The answer you are looking for is right in front of you, in the foods that you eat every day.

Food for Health is the ultimate nutritional guide to self sufficient health and well being. It will provide you with the tools to maximise your health or improve specific conditions using everyday foods. Whilst eating an 'optimum nutrition' diet will have the greatest effect upon your health, there's no need for an 'all or nothing' approach, and this book provides a range of options, from making simple dietary changes right through to following an optimum nutrition eating plan for your health condition. Whether you want to reduce the risk of familial conditions such as arthritis or diabetes, improve existing health conditions such as high cholesterol, or follow a diet to reduce inflammation, this book provides the know how.

Doctors and healthcare professionals may provide some guidance on how to adapt your diet to improve conditions such as indigestion or diabetes, especially with the increasing interest in lifestyle medicine, but the science of nutrition and how food affects our body is a specialist subject, so you are assured of the best advice from a qualified nutritionist or dietician. Details of how to find a qualified practitioner in your area are included in the help list in this book.

If you want to take greater control of your own health and learn how to be your own 'food doctor', then this is the book for you. Food for Health – The Essential Guide opens the door to a healthier way of life for you and your family through simple dietary changes all supported by research.

In each chapter you will find:

- A simple explanation of what each disease condition is
- Research and Information on foods which may help to improve the condition and ease its symptoms
- Tips on how to reduce your risk of developing certain health conditions
- Scientific research to support dietary and supplement recommendations

'If the doctors of today don't become nutritionists, the nutritionists will become the doctors of tomorrow.'

- Simple tips to help you make dietary changes – how to fit recommended foods into your diet, ways to maximize nutrient content and food swaps

- Information on therapeutic supplements, herbs and spices.

Recipes and seven-day eating plans for various disease conditions are included in Appendix A and Appendix B.

Whether you're ready to give your diet a complete overhaul or just looking for quick and easy ways to eat a healthier diet, you can choose a way of changing your diet that suits you:

- Quick changes – watch out for tick lists to show you how to fit more of a specific food into your diet

- Ready for a bit more – Aim to make more than one dietary change, and try the recipes as well

- Diet overhaul – follow one of the seven day eating plans.

Food for Health – The Essential Guide offers the ultimate guide to improving your health through diet – handed to you 'on a plate'! All you have to do is eat it!

'Let food be your medicine, and medicine be your food'

Hippocrates
AD390

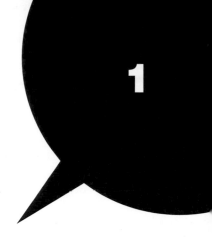

1

Food for a healthy heart

For over fifty years, dietary recommendations to reduce the risk of cardiovascular disease (CVD) have focused on reducing saturated fat intake, with additional recommendations to also limit dietary cholesterol intake. Despite this, 160,000 people die from heart and circulatory disease in the UK every year (Heart UK, 2018), and more recent research suggests that there is no connection between the intake of saturated fat and heart disease, and that other aspects of our diet are more likely to have an adverse effect upon the risk of cardiovascular disease. There are several simple dietary changes that can significantly improve cardiovascular health, postponing or even reducing the onset of degenerative heart disease and cardiovascular disease.

What is cardiovascular disease?

Cardiovascular disease is often characterized by a combination of high blood pressure, atherosclerosis ('furring up' of the arteries) and elevated cholesterol levels, but other factors may be involved. Although we commonly use the term 'heart disease', these conditions affect the blood vessels going to and from the heart (hence the term 'vascular'), as well as the blood vessels directly servicing the heart itself.

Hypertension

Hypertension is consistently high blood pressure. A 'normal' blood pressure reading is approximately 120/80, although this figure tends to increase from our mid-twenties as we age. The higher the blood pressure on the inside of the artery walls, the greater the likelihood of damage, and once damaged, substances are more likely to adhere to, and interact with, the endothelium on the inside of the blood vessels, causing atherosclerosis.

Atherosclerosis

This is the result of plaque formation inside the arteries; a build up of fats and cellular debris within the inner wall of the arteries, progressively thickening the endothelium (inner membrane of the artery). Damage caused by oxidized cholesterol or trans fats increases the migration of white blood cells, inflammatory proteins and clotting proteins to the area, creating a build up of plaque and narrowing the artery. Atherosclerotic plaques within the artery walls are formed mostly from fats and inflammatory cells. As cholesterol is a component of every cell in the human body, it has been suggested that more cholesterol is released from the liver and carried to the damaged area of an artery for new cell formation, creating the elevated cholesterol levels often found in conjunction with chronic inflammation (and cardiovascular disease).

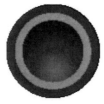

Normal artery

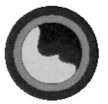

Plaque build-up in
artery wall

As plaque builds up, it reduces the space for blood to travel through, and this increases blood pressure, which creates even more damage to the artery walls. Once the smooth inner membrane of an artery is damaged, substances travelling in the blood stream are more likely to adhere to the roughened surface, worsening the atherosclerosis and narrowing the artery even more. Although hypertension (high blood pressure) and atherosclerosis are two separate conditions, they each cause the other.

Arteriosclerosis

This is a hardening of the artery walls often found alongside atherosclerosis. As our artery walls are made from the foods that we eat, the types of fats we consume and the balance of minerals such as calcium, magnesium, sodium and potassium affect how flexible our artery walls are. Our artery walls are partially formed from the fats that we eat – too many saturated or refined (hydrogenated or trans) fats create a rigid artery wall, whereas polyunsaturated fats, from fish and vegetable sources, promote flexibility. A diet high in sodium (salt) or calcium, or deficient in magnesium also contributes to less flexible, rigid artery walls that fail to 'give' when blood pressure increases, increasing the risk of damage. Damaged arteries may become progressively calcified over time. Smoking also contributes to arteriosclerosis.

Cholesterol

The cholesterol in our diet only provides approximately 20% of our cholesterol. We make the rest ourselves in the liver, and use it to form cell membranes, to make hormones, and to form bile for fat digestion, so a certain amount of cholesterol is required for good health. Although the level of LDL ('bad') cholesterol in the bloodstream increases the *risk* of developing cardiovascular disease, it is the preponderance of *small, dense LDL particles* and *oxidized* LDL cholesterol that seems to cause arterial wall damage, increasing inflammatory processes that contribute to plaque formation. The amount of cholesterol circulating in a healthy body is not the major causative factor of cardiovascular disease; factors such as oxidation, free radical damage and inflammation increase the risk of cardiovascular disease by affecting cholesterol metabolism. High levels of high density lipoprotein (HDL) 'good' cholesterol help to counteract high levels of 'bad' LDL cholesterol, as these lipoproteins (cholesterol carriers) transport cholesterol out of the blood stream and back to the liver, where it is used to form bile, which goes into the digestive tract. Once in the digestive tract, some of the cholesterol will be excreted in the stools.

'Patients with normal cholesterol levels have the same death rate as those with high cholesterol, suggesting that cholesterol only plays a partial role in heart disease.'

Reducing cholesterol intake has little effect on your cholesterol levels, and recent research has even suggested that saturated fat is not linked with an increased risk of cardiovascular events or death. However, your diet can have a major impact on blood lipid levels and the risk of cardiovascular disease. Rather than attempt to eat less cholesterol, or even reduce your saturated fat intake, it seems that the key may not be to simply eat less cholesterol or less saturated fat, but make dietary changes that will have the following effects:

- Reduce levels of free radicals and oxidized fats
- Increase anti-oxidant intake to reduce free radical damage and cholesterol oxidation
- Improve glucose metabolism in order to decrease inflammation and LDL oxidation, so reducing damage to artery walls.

As research shows conflicting opinion as to whether our cholesterol intake, fat intake and cholesterol levels actually cause heart disease, it is important to also consider the positive impact that various dietary changes will have upon other cardiovascular risk factors such as reducing overall weight and central obesity, reducing the risk of type 2 diabetes, metabolic syndrome and insulin resistance, and reducing oxidative stress in the body. All of these factors also increase the risk of cholesterol becoming oxidized and contributing to atherosclerotic plaques in the artery walls, heightening the risk of cardiovascular disease. So, if changing your diet can reduce these risk factors, you can reduce your risk of cardiovascular disease, regardless of the effect upon your cholesterol levels.

What does a heart-healthy diet look like?

There are a number of dietary changes that will reduce your risk of cardiovascular disease:

- You can reduce your overall fat, sugar and calorie intake to reduce the risk of abdominal obesity
- You can reduce your intake of processed fats (trans fats and hydrogenated fats) as these have a detrimental effect upon healthy cholesterol metabolism
- You can eat fats that will help to build healthy artery walls and provide a more favorable cholesterol metabolism
- You can eat more anti-oxidants to limit oxidation of fats and cholesterol
- You can reduce the amount of salt in your diet, which will reduce the risk of hypertension.

Limit sugars and refined carbohydrate foods

There is a connection between fat stored around the middle (central obesity), disturbed blood glucose regulation and high blood pressure; having all three is a condition called Metabolic Syndrome. Central obesity and insulin resistance are both powerful risk factors for cardiovascular disease; with increased adiposity around the middle, hepatic (liver) production of LDL increases, leading to elevated triglyceride levels and impaired LDL/HDL ratio. All these changes exert a significant pro-thrombotic and pro-inflammatory state. In their meta-analysis and review measuring the association between metabolic disease and cardiovascular disease, Mottillo *et al* (2010) reported a 2-fold increase in the risk of cardiovascular disease, stroke, and death from cardiovascular disease in those with metabolic syndrome.

The excess glucose from too many cakes, pastries, sweets, chocolate and white bread products causes high blood glucose levels and insulin resistance. Obesity and insulin resistance are both powerful risk factors for cardiovascular disease, and fat that is stored around the middle (central obesity) secretes inflammatory markers that increase blood pressure and cholesterol levels.

Reducing carbohydrate intake

Many experts are now suggesting that carbohydrate intake should not exceed 50% of total energy intake, and low carbohydrate diets such as paleo and ketogenic diets are on the increase. However, carbohydrate foods are useful for energy, fibre, essential vitamins, minerals and phytonutrients.

Follows these guidelines to get your carbohydrate intake right:

- ✓ Consume only small portions of whole grain carbohydrates, reducing portion sizes of starchy carbohydrates such as rice, pasta, noodles, bread, cereals and potatoes

- ✓ Fill up on non-starch carbohydrates such as fruits and vegetables

- ✓ Choose lower GI carbohydrates such as beans, lentils and oats for healthier glucose metabolism

- ✓ Avoid or limit foods with a high GI, particularly sugary foods and refined carbohydrates such as biscuits, cakes, muffins and pastries.

'An increased waist circumference has been positively associated with the use of sweeteners such as saccharin, aspartame and sucralose, and both fasting glucose and triglyceride values are positively associated with total sweetener consumption, so these should also be avoided.'

Tips to help you reduce the carbohydrate load of your meals

What to reduce	What to add in
Reduce your portion size of cereal to 35g or less	Add nuts or seeds, or low GI fruit – cherries, citrus fruits, apple, pear, cherries, prunes or strawberries...
Reduce your portion of rice to 60g or less	Add vegetables to the rice whilst it cooks, risotto-style. Pack it out with onions, garlic, frozen peas, peppers and sweet corn. Alternatively, cook the rice separately but add extra vegetables to the other part of your meal, packing out chili, curry or stroganoff with vegetables containing less starch and fewer calories.
Reduce your portion of pasta to 60g or less	Replace starchy pasta with water-rich aubergines, courgettes, tomatoes, red onions and garlic for a lower calorie and tastier Mediterranean style meal with added health benefits.
Eat fewer potatoes!	Swap potatoes for other vegetables. The bright colours of vegetables such as pumpkin, carrot, beetroot or broccoli denotes the high levels of phytonutrients in these foods, which all contain less starch and fewer calories than potatoes.

'An apple a day keeps the doctor away.'

Eating a low GI diet

It isn't just the amount of carbohydrate that we eat that can present a problem, but also the type of carbohydrate foods eaten. There is an increasing body of evidence linking elevated cholesterol levels and impaired cholesterol metabolism to a diet rich in refined carbohydrates. Such a diet, based upon white bread and bakery products, and a large amount of foods with a high glycaemic index (GI), causes problems with elevated blood glucose and glucose metabolism. Ravid et al (2008) illustrated that a high glucose concentration after a meal increases intestinal cholesterol absorption. A diet high in sugars and refined carbohydrates also contributes to conditions such as insulin resistance, metabolic syndrome and diabetes, and these conditions are all linked with increased levels of oxidative stress. Oxidative stress is linked with higher levels of oxidized cholesterol, and therefore linked with increased risk of cardiovascular disease.

How do high GI carbohydrates affect cardiovascular risk factors?

Excess carbohydrate intake or dysfunctional glucose metabolism seem to contribute to cardiovascular disease through a number of possible routes:

- High blood glucose increases LDL cholesterol
- High blood glucose enhances oxidation

- Increased fat deposition as excess calories are taken in is common in diets that are high in refined carbohydrate foods which fail to 'fill you up', prompting further eating

- Meals high in carbohydrate and/or foods with a high GI also incite a higher insulin release, promoting fat storage and reducing the breakdown of fats for energy, both of which contribute to visceral and abdominal weight gain 'around the middle'

- High glucose levels and central adiposity can both cause inflammation, which affects cells and causes insulin resistance. This disturbs glucose metabolism further and contributes to the onset of metabolic syndrome and Type 2 diabetes, and all the aforementioned factors resulting from these conditions that heighten the risk of cardiovascular disease.

Are you at risk?

Knowing your waist circumference or waist-hip ratio can help you to discover whether you are storing excess calories around the middle. Waist circumferences of over 88cm for women and over 102cm for men increase the risk of Type 2 diabetes and heart disease. Here are the recommended guidelines suggested by the NHS.

Waist circumference guidelines for women	Waist circumference guidelines for men
Ideal: less than 80cm (32 inches) High: 80cm to 88cm (32 to 35 inches Very high: more than 88cm (35 inches)	Ideal: less than 94cm (37 inches) High: 94cm to 102cm (37 to 40 inches) Very high: more than 102cm (40 inches)

(NHS, 2018).

For people of South Asian origin there is an even greater health risk linked with central obesity, with waist measurements of 80cm in women and 90cm in men putting health at risk. The Ashwell Shape Chart © below illustrates how your waist measurement might be affecting your health.

'Being 'apple shaped' increases your risk of poor cholesterol metabolism, heart disease and diabetes.'

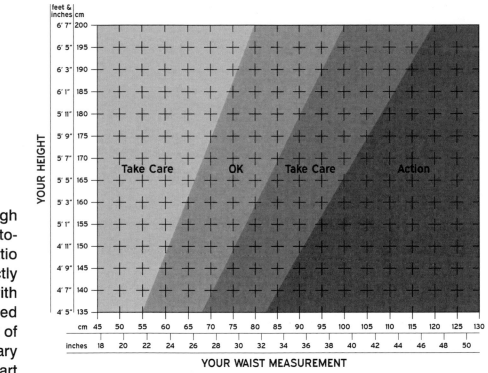

© Crown copyright. Source: Food Standards Agency.

'A high waist-to-hip ratio is directly linked with increased risk of coronary heart disease.'

Waist-hip ratio

Your waist-hip ratio compares the circumference of your waist to your hips – the more 'apple' shaped you are, the higher the health risks. To calculate your waist-hip ratio, simply divide your waist measurement by your hip measurement. For example, if your waist measurement was 80cm and your hips measured 110cm, your waist-hip ratio would be 0.72.

$$\frac{\text{Waist } 80}{\text{Hips } 110} = 0.72$$

Make sure that both measurements are either in inches or in centimeters.

Women	Men
Ideal: less than 0.8	Ideal: less than 0.90
Too high: 0.85 or more	Too high: 1 or more

Eat the right types of fats

Not all fats are bad: eating more fish and foods rich in polyunsaturated fats, such as nuts, and mono-unsaturated fats, such as olive oil or avocado, is actually linked with reduced cardiovascular risk. Saturated fats and trans fats make cell membranes rigid, therefore reducing the elasticity of artery walls and making them more at risk of damage. The types of unsaturated fats found in fish, vegetable oils, nuts and seeds help to form more flexible artery walls.

Oxidized dietary fats

Fats may become oxidized before they enter the body, through being heated, processed or exposed to prolonged light, and the 'healthy' polyunsaturated fats found in fish, nuts and seeds are more prone to oxidation than saturated fats found in meat and dairy produce. However, different types of fat seem to be metabolized differently in the body. Staprans et al (2005) found that consumption of oxidized linoleic acid (a polyunsaturated fat) only remained oxidized in chylomicrons immediately post-digestion, and were cleared from the body within 8 hours, with no increases in oxidized cholesterol.

Fats and cholesterol

A meta-analysis by Mensink and Katan (2003) measured the effect of dietary fats and carbohydrates on the ratio of total/HDL cholesterol, blood lipid levels and apolipoproteins, and found that the most beneficial changes were achieved by replacing saturated fats with unsaturated fats, reducing carbohydrate intake, and most importantly, reducing the intake of trans fatty acids. They also illustrated that different types of saturated fat (different length fatty acid chains) could have differing effects upon cholesterol and blood lipids, including some positive effects. It seems that not all saturated fats have a detrimental effect upon cholesterol metabolism and cardiovascular risk.

'A 2% absolute increase in energy intake from trans fat has been associated with a 23% increase in cardiovascular risk.'

Remig et al, Department of Human Nutrition, Kansas State University, USA.

The effects of consuming saturated fat upon cholesterol levels

A meta-analysis involving 21 studies and 347,747 subjects to determine the association of dietary saturated fat with risk of coronary heart disease, stroke, and cardiovascular disease showed no association between saturated fat intake and increased risk of heart disease, stroke or cardiovascular disease (Siri-Tarino *et al*, 2010). The PURE study (Dehghan *et al*, 2017) reviewed the food intake of 135,335 individuals in 18 countries against total mortality and cardiovascular events. They found that total fat intake was associated with a lower risk of overall mortality, higher saturated fat intake was associated with lower risk of stroke, and total fat, saturated and unsaturated fats were not significantly associated with risk of heart attack or cardiovascular disease mortality. However, higher carbohydrate intake was associated with an increased risk of total mortality, although not with the risk of cardiovascular disease or cardiovascular disease mortality.

They suggested that global dietary guidelines should be reconsidered in light of these findings.

However, a review of the effects of fat intake on cholesterol levels and development of cardiovascular disease by Hooper *et al* (2011) illustrated a 14% reduction in cardiovascular events by reducing saturated fat intake, but as neither total or LDL cholesterol were reduced, or HDL levels increased by eating less saturated fat, this result may be down to other effects such as reduced central obesity and fewer inflammatory markers, rather than any direct effect from lower saturated fat intake, or upon circulating cholesterol levels.

Coconut oil

In the last few years coconut oil has been touted as being a 'cure-all' fat, with claims to reduce cardiovascular disease, diabetes and even aid weight loss. The interesting thing about these claims is that coconut oil contains more saturated fat than butter! A review by Eyres *et al* (2016) illustrated that coconut oil generally raised total and LDL cholesterol more than unsaturated plant oils, but to a lesser extent than butter. Khaw *et al* (2018) compared the effects of consuming 50g coconut oil in comparison to 50g olive oil or butter on blood lipid profile, weight, fat distribution and metabolic markers after four weeks, with the following findings:

- Butter increased LDL levels more than coconut oil and olive oil
- Butter significantly increased triglyceride/HDL ratio and non-HDL levels compared with coconut and olive oil

- There were no significant differences in changes in LDL cholesterol between coconut oil and olive oil

- Coconut oil significantly increased HDL compared with butter and olive oil

- There were no significant differences in changes in weight, BMI, central adiposity, fasting blood glucose or blood pressure in any of the three intervention groups.

So it seems that two different saturated fats (butter and coconut oil) have different effects on blood lipids, and the blood lipid effects of coconut oil are more comparable to those of olive oil, which is a predominantly monounsaturated fat.

Hence, it cannot be claimed that saturated fats will increase cardiovascular risk, as it appears that the differing fatty acid profiles in saturated fats have different metabolic effects in the human body, and trials are still reporting inconsistent results. Further research into the effects of different types of fatty acid, rather than different types of dietary fat, are required.

Whether the small decreases in total and LDL cholesterol and triglycerides was the reason for reduced cardiovascular events shown in some trials, or whether the reduction and/or modified fat intake reduced cardiovascular disease via another mechanism, such as lower intra-abdominal obesity and reduced inflammatory response, it is worth making these changes to your diet. Research is still providing conflicting results linking fat intake to cholesterol levels, but changing the type of fat you eat does seem to reduce cardiovascular disease via some mechanism.

Moderating your fat intake based upon the evidence

Although much of the research on the effects of fat intake on both cholesterol levels and cardiovascular disease shows conflicting results, these adaptations will help you to reduce your risk of cardiovascular disease through one or more mechanisms.

Saturated fat

Whether saturated fat increases total and LDL cholesterol or not, eating too much will contribute to obesity and Type 2 diabetes, which are both additional risk factors for cardiovascular disease. Saturated fat is not a preferred type of fat for use in the formation of the artery endothelium; if used for this task, it increases the rigidity of the

'The effects of different dietary fats on lipid profiles, metabolic markers and health outcomes may vary not just because of the general classification of fatty acids (saturated or unsaturated), but possibly according to the foods they occur in, and the different profiles in individual fatty acids.'

Khaw et al, 2018.

artery walls, increasing the risk of arteriosclerosis, hypertension and atherosclerosis. Therefore, with all things considered, it is still recommended that you consume more natural unsaturated fats than foods rich in saturated fat.

As more recent research illustrates that saturated fat may not contribute to cardiovascular disease, it makes sense to include eggs, fresh meat, and organic dairy foods in your diet, and limit the following foods that contain saturated fat, but also have additional health risks associated with them.

Foods to limit

- Cured and smoked meats (bacon, salami, chorizo etc.)
- Confectionary such as cakes, pastries, biscuits, ice cream and chocolate.

'The NHS recommends that we eat at least two portions of fish a week, of which one portion should be oily fish.'

Unsaturated fats

Eating polyunsaturated and monounsaturated fats may help to reduce overall cholesterol and LDL cholesterol, increase HDL cholesterol levels, and improve your total/HDL ratio. However, this may not have a direct effect upon cardiovascular disease because of the effect upon LDL or HDL cholesterol, but may enhance the flexibility of the artery endothelium, reducing the risk of the thickening or hardening of the arteries, and hypertension. Eating more fish and nuts (rich in polyunsaturated fats) and foods containing mono-unsaturated fats, such as olive oil or avocado, has been linked with reduced cardiovascular risk. However, these fats are at greater risk of oxidation prior to consumption, so limit heating and exposure to light, and avoid processed unsaturated fats (trans and hydrogenated), found in some margarines and sauces.

Oxidation of unsaturated fats

Polyunsaturated vegetables oils such as sunflower or safflower oil are not as healthy when heated or processed, as oxygen can easily combine with them. These oxygen atoms are only loosely connected to the rest of the fat, and are likely to separate from the fat once in the body, becoming something called a free radical. As the oxygen attaches to other molecules or cells, this causes free radical damage in the body, so it is best to consume these oils directly from their natural source (nuts and seeds) or use the oils cold as a salad dressing.

Monounsaturated fat is found mostly in plant foods and oils, and contains only one double bond in each fatty acid chain. Only having one double bond limits the risk of oxidation in comparison to polyunsaturated fatty acids, which have several double bonds. This is why olive oil is still considered to be a good choice to cook with, particularly at lower temperatures. Coconut oil, which is highly saturated, has a lower risk of oxidation during heating.

Foods rich in polyunsaturated fat

- Fish
- Nuts
- Seeds
- Vegetable oils

Foods rich in monounsaturated fat

- Avocados
- Nuts
- Seeds
- Olives
- Olive oil

Tips to eat more fish

- Swap a breakfast fry up for kippers
- Enjoy kedgeree or sardines on toast for brunch or lunch
- Add salmon or tuna to sandwiches instead of cheese, egg or meat
- Swap meat for fish in at least two evening meals.

White fish such as cod or haddock do contain the heart-healthy long chain fatty acids, but as they store more fat in their liver rather than in their flesh, you have to consume cod liver oil capsules to get a rich source of fish oils. Although oily fish store fat in their flesh, the essential oils are mostly lost during the canning process, so tinned fish will contain lower levels of fatty acids similar to the levels found in non-oily fish.

'Daily fish consumption reduces overall mortality by 16% and incidence of death due to myocardial infarction (heart attack) by 24%.' Yzebe and Lievre, Lyon Hospitals, France.

Olive oil – cardio-protective properties

The Mediterranean-style diet has been repeatedly linked with a decreased risk of cardiovascular disease due to reduced cholesterol and blood pressure measurements, improved glucose metabolism, and reduced damage and inflammation in artery walls. Although this is due to many dietary factors, one plus point is the consumption of monounsaturated fats rather than saturated fats. These types of fats are found mostly in plant foods and oils such as avocados, nuts, seeds and olive oil. In 2014, the Food and Drug Administration (USA) determined that a minimum daily intake of 17.5 grams of unheated monounsaturated fatty acids from olive oil (2 tablespoons) exerts a positive effect on reduction of coronary heart disease.

How to add heart-healthy fats to your diet

- Dip your bread in olive oil rather than spreading butter on it
- Add avocado or vegetable oil dressings to salads rather than processed sauces
- Cook with olive oil or coconut oil
- Snack on nuts and seeds rather than biscuits and cakes.

A final word on fats

In some trials, better results were seen when the type of fat rather than the overall intake of fat was adjusted. However, all types of fat contain approximately 9 calories per gram and will contribute to weight gain, so to reduce the risk of obesity and Type 2 diabetes – which both independently increase the risk of heart disease – limit overall fat intake to approximately 30% of your daily caloric intake.

Avoid high fat foods by checking the total fat content on nutrition labels.
High fat foods contain more than 17.5g of total fat per 100g
Low fat foods contain 3g or less of total fat per 100g
Low fat drinks contain less than 1.5g of fat per 100ml

If your individual genetic metabolism does respond by increasing your total or LDL cholesterol in response to fat intake, then it is worth reducing your overall fat intake. Elevated cholesterol in itself may not present a problem, but higher levels of LDL cholesterol – particularly the small, dense type of LDL particle – can increase the risk of entry into the artery walls and increase oxidation.

Increase anti-oxidant intake with more fruit and vegetables

Fruits and vegetables offer several benefits in a heart-healthy diet:

- Many of these foods are rich in anti-oxidants, helping to reduce oxidation

- They are lower in calories and fats, reducing abdominal obesity and Type 2 diabetes

- Many fruits and vegetables are rich in potassium and naturally low in sodium (salt), and can help to maintain a healthy blood pressure

- Fruits and vegetables contain types of fibre known to help lower cholesterol levels.

Rich in anti-oxidants

Oxidation is a serious contributor to cardiovascular disease. However, it can be reduced by nutrients called anti-oxidants, and several large-scale studies have illustrated that a high anti-oxidant intake benefits arterial health. Phytonutrients (plant nutrients) known as flavonoids and proanthocyanidins have been found to have a powerful anti-oxidant effect.

For example, tomatoes contain a nutrient called lycopene, which has been found to have several cardio-protective properties:

- It has a high anti-oxidant content

- It regulates cholesterol synthesis

- It stimulates the breakdown on 'bad' LDL cholesterol

- Low blood levels of lycopene have been linked with a higher incidence of death from heart disease.

'Hertog et al (1993) illustrated that risk of death from cardiovascular disease was 68% lower in those consuming the highest amount of flavonoids.'

Fruit and vegetables can reduce blood pressure

Many large population studies show a positive association between fruit and vegetable consumption and decreased risk of heart disease. One of the ways that fruit and vegetables can help to reduce the risk of heart disease is by lowering blood pressure. One study reports that eating fruit and vegetables can reduce systolic and diastolic blood pressure by 6.8 and 2.1 mmHg respectively over a year (Moore *et al*, 2008).

Fruits and vegetables reduce cholesterol

Regular consumption of fruit and vegetables can help to reduce your risk of heart disease through lowering cholesterol levels. Positive cholesterol-lowering results are repeatedly associated with apple, garlic and other foods such as chicory and asparagus. It is the fibre and the phytosterols in these foods that are the active ingredients responsible for the cholesterol lowering benefits.

The cholesterol in our bloodstream comes from two sources – cholesterol that we eat in foods such as egg yolks, and the cholesterol that our liver makes. Cholesterol is carried in bile from the liver and squirted from the gall bladder into the duodenum (small intestine). Both types of cholesterol end up in the digestive tract, where plant sterols (phytosterols) compete with cholesterol for absorption, blocking the amount of dietary cholesterol that can be absorbed back into the body. In addition, fibre binds with cholesterol and carries it out of the body in the faeces.

'The risk for cardiovascular disease among vegetarian populations is consistently 20% to 35% below that for omnivore populations.'
Key *et al*, Cancer Epidemiology Unit, Oxford, UK.

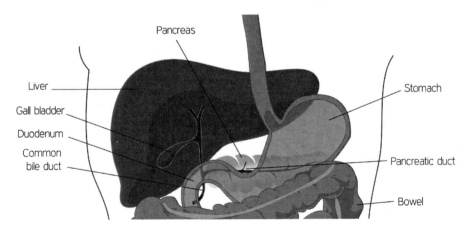

Eating more high fibre foods can help to reduce the risk of cardiovascular disease in a number of other ways:

- Fibre travels on to the large intestine and creates favorable by-products during fermentation which re-enter the blood stream and lower blood lipid levels

- Fibre intake increases satiety (the feeling of fullness) and helps with weight control – central obesity is associated with higher levels of LDL and elevated triglyceride levels

- Fibre helps to regulate glucose absorption and blood sugar control, diminishing the development of insulin resistance and metabolic syndrome, which both increase the risk of cardiovascular disease

- Poor blood glucose metabolism causes oxidative stress, which is known to be detrimental to cholesterol metabolism and increases plaque formation.

As obesity and diabetes seem to increase the amount of oxidized cholesterol and heighten the risk of heart disease, dietary changes that help to reduce the risk of these diseases are definite 'must-do's!

Foods rich in fibre include:

- Fruit and vegetables

- Beans and pulses

- Whole grains

- Nuts and seeds.

Many fruits and vegetables contain fibre that will help to lower cholesterol, but inulin is a type of fibre that is really effective at carrying cholesterol out of the body. Inulin is found in foods such as garlic, onion, asparagus, Jerusalem artichoke and chicory. The beta glucan fibre in oats is also very effective at reducing cholesterol levels; its effectiveness is so evident that several regulatory bodies have approved a health claim on the cholesterol-lowering effects of oat β-glucan at levels of 3g/day, allowing this information to appear on certain oat-based food products. Beta-glucan is a type of soluble fibre, also found in barley, and it binds with cholesterol (and bile acids), taking them out of the body with the faeces.

Fenugreek seeds

In addition to the beneficial cholesterol-lowering effect of the fibre in fenugreek seeds, they contain compounds called saponins that inhibit cholesterol absorption in the intestines, and also reduce hepatic cholesterol production. In a 2009 clinical trial, 24 Type 2 diabetic patients were given 10g/day powdered fenugreek seeds mixed with yoghurt or soaked in hot water for 8 weeks. Fasting blood sugar, triglycerides and VLDL decreased significantly (25%, 30% and 30.6% respectively) after taking the fenugreek seeds soaked in hot water (Kassiain et al, 2009).

'Over five weeks consuming beta glucan from oats added to a juice drink, total cholesterol reduced by 4.8% and LDL cholesterol reduced by 7.7%.'

Naumann et al, Maastricht University, Netherlands.

Phytosterols

Phytosterols reduce cholesterol by competing for intestinal absorption with both dietary and biliary (from the liver/gall bladder) cholesterol, causing a 30 – 50% reduction in cholesterol absorption. Anything that is not absorbed into the blood stream or lymphatic system during digestion (therefore remaining in the gastro-intestinal tract) proceeds on to the large intestine and leaves the body as faeces. Consuming 1.5-1.8 g/day of plant sterols or stanols can reduce cholesterol absorption by 30-40%, and 2.2 g/day of plant sterols has been shown to reduce cholesterol absorption by 60%. With less cholesterol circulating in the blood stream, cells are stimulated to take up more cholesterol, resulting in increased clearance of circulating LDL. Although the decreased cholesterol absorption due to phytosterol intake also stimulates increased cholesterol synthesis in the liver, the net result is generally a reduction in serum LDL cholesterol concentration.

Jenkins *et al* (2005) reported an average reduction in LDL cholesterol of 30% in participants following a diet including soy protein, almonds, oats, barley, psyllium husk fibre, okra and aubergine, and 1g of plant sterols daily from an enriched margarine. This reduction is not significantly different from the effects of statin drugs. However, the average LDL reduction with the same diet over one year, researched by Jenkins *et al* again, was only 13%, probably due to reduced dietary adherence, although one third of the participants did still have more than a 20% reduction in LDL levels.

Ostlund *et al* illustrated that removing the phytosterols from corn oil increased cholesterol absorption by 38% (2002) and removing phytosterols from wheat germ increased cholesterol absorption back into the body from the gut by 43% (2003), proving that eating phytosterol-rich foods really makes a difference to the amount of cholesterol that you absorb. However, one study (Alphonse *et al*, 2017) illustrated that plant sterol consumption failed to reduce LDL-cholesterol concentrations despite showing a 6% reduction in cholesterol absorption. There was an over-compensatory reciprocal increase in cholesterol synthesis after reduced cholesterol absorption when plant sterols were consumed, so individual variability in cholesterol metabolism may impact plasma lipid responses to dietary sterols in some healthy individuals.

Increasing your phytosterol intake

Consuming more natural phytosterol-rich foods in your diet will help to lower your cholesterol, so make the following changes:

- Snack on nuts (especially almonds) instead of biscuits, sweets or chocolate

- Eat whole grains rather than refined white flour products, and include oats in your diet

- Include more pulses and legumes in your diet

- Use unrefined vegetable oils or coconut oil instead of refined margarine spreads

- Swap minced beef for soya mince, or use soya products such as tofu, soya yoghurt and soya milk.

Phytosterol-enhanced foods

Plant sterols have been repeatedly proven to lower overall and low density lipoprotein (LDL) cholesterol, although the effects are enhanced by combining sterol-enriched foods with a healthy diet.

Reduction in cholesterol from using margarines with plant sterols added	Reduction in cholesterol from using enriched margarines plus eating more vegetables, fruit, soya and nuts.
Total cholesterol ⬇ 10% LDL cholesterol ⬇ 14%	Total cholesterol ⬇ 22.34% LDL cholesterol ⬇ 29.71%

(Buckley et al, 2007)

Important facts about phytosterols

It was previously thought that doses higher than 2 – 5g/day did not seem to substantially improve the cholesterol-lowering effects of plant sterols or stanols, but recent studies suggest a continuous dose–response effect in lowering LDL. A review of five trials demonstrated a linear dose-effect relationship, with the greatest LDL lowering outcome, 18%, achieved with a daily intake of 9 to 10g of plant stanols, with no reports of adverse effects.

- Reductions are likely to be greater in those with higher baseline (starting) levels of LDL cholesterol

- Reductions with phytosterol-enriched foods are greater in older adults

- The average cholesterol-lowering effect of plant sterols and stanols is a reduction in total or LDL cholesterol of 10 – 11%).

'For a healthy-heart diet, eat porridge made with soya milk and added nuts, seeds and fruit for breakfast, a large salad with chicory, onion and asparagus at lunchtime, and fish with broccoli and garlic-roasted squash and carrots for dinner.'

Phytosterols may also, as a lipid, potentially contribute to atherosclerosis, but their absorption rate is so low this is not considered to be a risk factor. After absorption into the intestinal cells, phytosterols are actively excreted back into the intestinal lumen.

How much will I need to consume to make a difference?

0.8-1.0g/day is the lowest dose that results in clinically significant LDL cholesterol reductions of at least 5%. A healthy diet provides approximately 160 – 400mg (0.16 – 0.4g) of phytosterols daily, and to sustain benefits from phytosterols, you need to consume at least 1g daily. If you are consuming phytosterol-enriched foods, you can follow the food manufacturer's guidelines as to how much of their products you need to consume to get up to 2g of sterols or stanols daily. This is usually equivalent to 1 yoghurt drink or 2-3 servings of spread, milk or yoghurt.

A down side to phytosterol-enriched foods

Although plant sterols have been proven to lower cholesterol, they can also reduce the absorption of some fat-soluble vitamins such as beta-carotene and vitamin E. As these anti-oxidants help to reduce the oxidation of LDL cholesterol, this is an important consideration when consuming phytosterol-enriched foods. Phytosterols or stanols can reduce the blood concentration of beta-carotene levels by 25% and vitamin E by 8%. If you don't have high cholesterol, you shouldn't be consuming phytosterol-enhanced foods, as these may reduce your cholesterol level too much, as well as reducing blood anti-oxidant levels. Children and women who are pregnant or breastfeeding should not regularly eat foods with added phytosterols. The National Heart Foundation in Australia recommend a limited consumption of added plant sterols or stanols, and advise consumption of at least one serving of carotenoid-rich foods daily to maintain carotene levels for those consuming functional foods with added plant sterols.

Carotenoid-rich foods

- Carrots
- Sweet potato
- Squash and pumpkin
- Peaches and apricots
- Green leafy vegetables.

Foods containing Vitamin E – an important anti-oxidant for cardiovascular health

- Snack on nuts and seeds, especially Brazil nuts, almonds and hazelnuts
- Drizzle high quality, cold vegetable oils on to salads
- Add pine nuts or sunflower seeds to salads and stir fries
- Add wheat germ to cereals or yoghurts
- Add avocado to salad sandwiches, salads and wraps.

Ways to consume phytosterols

1 Swap butter or margarine for a spread enriched with plant sterols/stanols
2 Swap full fat yoghurts to phytosterol-enriched or soya yoghurts (which contain natural phytosterols)
3 Choose milk enriched with phytosterols or use soya milk
4 Eat plenty of high fibre fruit, vegetables, oats and beans rich in natural phytosterols
5 Drink phytosterol-enriched juices
6 Eat soya protein – soya milk, soya beans, soya yoghurts, tofu...
7 Snack on nuts and seeds.

Make sure you make healthy changes

As elevated cholesterol levels often occur with increased body weight, eating large amounts of margarine is not the best way to consume phytosterols to reduce cholesterol, as you would be simultaneously increasing your intake of a processed fat and calories, which may increase your weight. Aim to get phytosterols from foods that naturally contain them, then top up with enriched juices or yoghurts, or consider a phytosterol supplement. Phytosterol-enriched foods can be a useful, although sometimes expensive, adjunct to your diet, as they add an additional amount of plant sterols to your daily consumption. However, you should not rely upon these functional foods, but make healthy changes to your overall diet and lifestyle for maximum benefits.

'You may benefit from adding phytosterols to your diet if your total cholesterol is over 5mmol/l or if you have LDL ('bad' cholesterol) of over 2.6mmol/l.'

Garlic – cardiovascular superfood

Both onion and garlic were used in ancient Egypt, Greece and Italy for heart disease. Garlic contains a number of sulphur compounds that provide its pungent odour but are also extremely beneficial for our health. In addition to immune-supportive, anti-tumour and anti-carcinogenic benefits, garlic has several cardiovascular properties:

- It 'thins' the blood, making it less likely to clot
- It reduces blood pressure by vasodilating (widening) blood vessels
- It reduces triglycerides (fats) in the blood
- It contains inulin fibre that helps to reduce 'bad' LDL cholesterol.

'Adding raw garlic to uncrushed micro-waved garlic re-instates its anti-clotting ability.' Cavagnaro et al, Journal of Agricultural and Food Chemistry.

For allicin, one of the main therapeutic compounds in garlic, to be most active, the garlic should be crushed and left for up to ten minutes, and eaten raw. Crushing, slicing or pressing garlic activates the enzyme that forms the active compounds that have 'heart-healthy properties', some of which are still viable with up to six minutes of boiling or oven roasting garlic at 200°C, so garlic still retains some therapeutic properties with light cooking if it is crushed, and the loss of anti-clotting properties can be offset by increasing the amount eaten.

To enjoy the heart healthy benefits of garlic...

- Eat crushed, sliced or grated garlic raw
- Crush, slice, grate or press the garlic and leave for up to ten minutes to allow the enzyme alliinase form the active compounds
- If cooking garlic, crush it first, allow it to rest to maximise the amount of anti-clotting sulphur compounds to form, then cook moderately for no more than six minutes
- Add a little raw garlic to microwaved uncrushed garlic to re-instate its anti-clotting properties.

Although garlic capsules are less pungent, their efficacy relies on the supplement preparation. Where the active ingredients of garlic are concentrated within a garlic capsule, cardiovascular benefits are noted. Sobenin et al (2009) reported a reduction of 7mm Hg in systolic blood pressure and 3.8 mm Hg in diastolic blood pressure after participants took time-release garlic powder tablets for eight weeks.

Alcohol and cardiovascular disease
– the red wine paradox

France and other Mediterranean countries have a lower incidence of cardiovascular 'events', despite the same risk factors such as diabetes, high blood pressure and elevated cholesterol levels. Data from at least twenty countries in Europe, North America, Asia and Australia shows a 20 to 40% lower incidence of coronary heart disease amongst those that consume a moderate amount of alcohol, in comparison with non-drinkers or heavy drinkers. There appears to be a J shaped relationship between alcohol consumption and heart disease, with increased risk of heart disease in those consuming more than two drinks daily, or none at all. In a sixteen year study, Tverdal *et al* (2017) found that teetotallers had higher risk of dying from cardiovascular disease than alcohol consumers, and wine had the most favourable outcomes.

It seems that despite a similar amount of arterial damage caused by fatty plaques and high blood pressure in those that consume alcohol, this damage is somehow offset by having a greater degree of 'relaxation' in the artery walls, lower levels of inflammation and less blood clotting. The most favorable outcome is from consuming red wine – this is partly due to substances in the grapes used to make the wine. Polyphenols, particularly resveratrol, contribute to cardiovascular protection mainly through antioxidant properties, exerting beneficial effects on endothelial dysfunction in the artery walls, and also reducing hypertension, dyslipidemia and metabolic diseases such as insulin resistance. It is also suggested that the alcohol (ethanol) itself appears to have a relaxing effect upon the artery walls that makes them less liable to damage from elevated blood pressure, as other alcoholic beverages, such as beer, also show reduced cardiovascular risk from consuming moderate amounts (1 – 2 units daily).

Drinking one to two alcoholic beverages daily can increase your 'good' cholesterol (high density lipoprotein) by approximately 12%. The 'good' cholesterol reduces the amount of 'bad' cholesterol (LDL) in the blood stream and limits the risk of atherosclerosis. In addition to this, the anti-oxidants in red wine limit oxidation of LDL and other fats, further reducing plague formation.

'Several studies show that the active component responsible for reduced cardiovascular disease is the polyphenols present in red wine, and the majority of research shows more positive results with wines from areas of south western France and the Mediterranean.'

'Patients with cardiovascular disease received red grape extract or placebo... after one hour, dilation (relaxation) of the brachial artery was enhanced 70% for the red grape extract group'.

Lekakis et al, Department of Cardiology, University General Hospital, Greece.

However, although a small amount of alcohol may reduce heart disease, consuming any more than one to two drinks daily is detrimental to good health. But if you do drink, it seems a good idea to limit consumption to one to two drinks daily, have a few days alcohol-free each week, and drink red wine as your chosen tipple!

Hypertension and salt

High salt (sodium chloride) consumption has been linked with hypertension, and a diet low in salt and high in fruit and vegetables has been proven to significantly reduce blood pressure. Fruit and vegetables are naturally low in sodium and rich in potassium, a mineral that helps to counteract the effects of sodium in the body.

Ways to reduce salt intake

- Stop adding salt to cooking
- Don't add salt to your food
- Check food labels for high salt or sodium content
- Avoid high salt foods such as marmite, anchovies, salted crisps and nuts
- Watch out for high salt foods that don't necessarily taste salty, such as cheese, bread and pizza
- Eat plenty of potassium-rich foods to counteract the effects of sodium – fill up on fruit and vegetables.

The NHS currently recommends limiting your salt intake to 6g daily, but some food labels list sodium rather than salt content. You can calculate the amount of salt in a food by multiplying the sodium content by 2.5. For example, if a portion of food contains 0.8g sodium, it will contain about 2g of salt.

The effects of caffeine

Caffeine, found in coffee, tea, some fizzy drinks and chocolate, makes our adrenal glands produce the hormone adrenaline. One of the effects of adrenaline is that it increases blood pressure through the effect of temporary narrowing of the small arteries in the body – this increase in blood pressure results in the kidneys producing more urine in an attempt to reduce blood (water) volume in the body to lower blood pressure, through the diuretic effects of caffeine.

'Start checking the salt content on tinned and packaged foods and choose low salt products. A high salt food contains more than 1.5g of salt per 100g (or 0.6g sodium per 100g), and a low salt food contains 0.3g salt or less per 100g (or 0.1g sodium).'

Adrenaline increases the amount of glucose and fats in the blood stream for energy – but think what you are usually doing when drinking a cup of tea or coffee... not exercising and using up this energy! Circulating fatty acids that aren't used for energy increase the risk of oxidation and contribution to atherosclerotic plaques on arterial walls, worsening any existing build up of fatty deposits, which in turn can increase blood pressure further. However, it is still unclear how consistent increase of blood pressure from drinking caffeinated beverages affects long-term cardiovascular health, particularly if hypertension or atherosclerosis already exists. Although drinking coffee increases blood pressure, Buscemi *et al,* (2010), found that total caffeine intake from drinking coffee, green tea or Oolong tea was associated with a reduced risk of death from cardiovascular disease. Chei *et al* (2017) reviewed several large health studies and the relationship between hypertension and caffeine intake. They found that drinking either less than one cup of coffee weekly or more than three cups daily had lower risk than drinking one cup a day. Caffeine may account for increased risk of hypertension in daily tea drinkers and in those who drank one cup of coffee a day. The inverse U-shaped association with coffee suggests that at higher doses, other ingredients in coffee may offset the effect of caffeine and confer blood pressure benefits.

Supplements to help

Fish oils

Fish oils in the diet and from supplementation have long been associated with a healthy heart and cardiovascular system. Many double-blind trials have demonstrated that fish oil supplements containing eicosapentanoic acid (EPA) and docosahexanoic acid (DHA) lower triglyceride levels. Fish oil supplementation has also been shown to reduce blood pressure, but the amounts often used in research trials are in excess of 3000mg (3g) EPA/DHA daily – that is the actual amount of EPA/DHA and not the total amount of fish oil in a typical 500mg or 1g capsule, and taking this amount of fish oil in supplement form is not always practical or sustainable. Fish oils are also associated with slowing down progression of arterial plaque formation, and decreasing cardiovascular events such as heart attack and stroke, so even if you don't supplement the amount used in research trials, it is a worthy supplement to consider.

Vitamin E

Vitamin E has several cardio-protective benefits, largely due to its anti-oxidant properties, which help to prevent cholesterol becoming oxidized and contributing to atherosclerosis, thrombosis, stroke and heart attacks. Some forms of vitamin E reduce liver production of cholesterol. It has been cited as the most potent anti-oxidant to reduce LDL cholesterol, reduce the oxidation of LDL cholesterol, and also block the actions of oxidized LDL cholesterol. Although earlier studies reported vitamin E supplementation reducing heart disease by 41%, and a 40% decrease in cholesterol oxidation after participants took 800IU of vitamin E daily for three months (Jialal and Grundy, 1992), other human trials have shown mixed results.

There are eight forms of vitamin E, four types of tocopherols and four types of tocotrienols. One human trial conducted by Yuen *et al* (2011) compared the effects of 300mg/day soya bean oil (rich in tocopherols) with 300mg/day of mixed tocotrienols from palm oil. After six months, total cholesterol decreased by 10.8% and LDL cholesterol decreased by 17.4% in the mixed tocotrienols group compared to the soya bean group. The differing actions of these types of vitamin E may explain the mixed results on lowering oxidized cholesterol in human trials. Tocotrienols inhibit the enzyme HMG-CoA reductase, which is involved in a pathway in the liver that synthesizes cholesterol, so this type of vitamin E may also be able to reduce blood cholesterol levels in the same way as statins do.

LDL can be oxidized by free radicals, by reactive oxygen species, and by lipoxygenase enzymes and cytochrome P450. Vitamin E only blocks free radical oxidation, so if oxidation through other means is high, this would interfere with the overall mean reduction in oxidized LDL. It also appears that vitamin E can only reduce oxidation early on, which may explain why Tang *et al* (2014) showed that vitamin E inhibits early but not advanced atherosclerotic lesion in ApoE mice. In en-vitro (test-tube) and animal studies, cholesterol is oxidized in the experiment just before vitamin E is administered, so the vitamin E is effective. In humans, LDL oxidation occurs over time, so much of the damage has already occurred before vitamin E is supplemented in trials. However, vitamin E can be used to prevent oxidation occurring in the first place.

Vitamin C

Vitamin C may also reduce heart disease by protecting LDL cholesterol from oxidative damage and from reducing cholesterol LDL levels. Use at least 100 mg per day to reduce LDL oxidation – some experts suggest using up to 1g (1000mg) daily. Siavash and Amini (2014) found that vitamin C supplementation increased HDL (good) cholesterol levels more than fibrate cholesterol medication (Gemfibrozil) in Type 2 diabetic patients, but did not reduce total cholesterol or triglycerides. Vitamin E works in conjunction with Vitamin C, the effects of each vitamin increased by the other, so a supplement containing both of these anti-oxidants is a good idea.

Vitamin B3 (Niacin)

Niacin has been shown to increase HDL levels, reduce VLDL and significantly reduce atherogenic sub-types of lipoprotein(a), and can also lower overall cholesterol and increase HDL cholesterol better than certain prescription drugs. It may also improve arterial endothelial function and reduce inflammation. Studies on niacin therapy have been almost universally favorable for lowering cholesterol, but Batuca *et al* (2017) found that the rise in HDL cholesterol is not matched with a corresponding increase in antioxidant capacity, which is why niacin (and other lipid lowering agents) may not reduce cardiovascular risk. It is thought this is due to the aApoA-I antibodies that appear with this therapy. High intakes of niacin can cause facial flushing, headaches or stomachache, or more severe effects in some cases, and may increase the risk of muscle damage if taken in conjunction with statins. Delayed-release 'non-blushing' forms of niacin are recommended if you are taking high doses.

Niacin not only lowers LDL cholesterol and raises HDL cholesterol, but it also appears to reduce the thickness of artery walls. A study comparing the effects of niacin with the drug Ezetimibe showed that those taking niacin had a significant reduction in artery thickness (therefore improving cardiovascular health), while those taking Ezetimibe experienced an increase in arterial thickness.

Magnesium

Magnesium has been shown to lower blood pressure and reduce occurrence of arrhythmias. Some, but not all, trials show that 350mg – 500mg of magnesium can lower blood pressure, and is particularly effective in people who are taking potassium-depleting diuretics, which deplete magnesium.

Co-Enzyme Q10 (CoQ10)

Some trials have reported that supplementation with CoQ10 can significantly decrease blood pressure in people with hypertension. Much of this research has used 100 mg of CoQ10 per day for at least ten weeks. One randomized controlled trial demonstrated improved functional capacity, a reduction in major adverse cardiovascular events and improved mortality with CoQ10 supplementation in patients with heart failure.

Statins work by inhibiting an enzyme that manufactures cholesterol in the liver. However, this also affects the production of co-enzyme Q10. Co-enzyme Q10 is found in virtually all cell membranes and, amongst many other functions, is essential for energy production in the body's cells. Together with Vitamin E, CoQ10 helps to protect LDL cholesterol from oxidation, so although statins may reduce the amount of cholesterol produced, they may also increase the oxidation of LDL cholesterol through lower CoQ10 levels, which is a greater risk factor for atherosclerosis and cardiovascular disease than the amount of circulating LDL cholesterol.

People with high cholesterol levels tend to have lower levels of CoQ10, and its natural production in the body also declines with age. There is no evidence that taking Co-enzyme Q10 will be beneficial to cholesterol levels, but as statins reduce levels of CoQ10, supplementing with this anti-oxidant will normalize levels in the body and may reduce side effects caused by statins such as muscle pain. Research has found reductions in oxidative stress in patients with coronary artery disease taking 150mg of CoQ10 daily. However, you should always consult your doctor if you experience any side effects from medication, and let them know if you are considering taking a CoQ10 supplement.

Chromium

Brewer's yeast, which contains up to 60mcg of absorbable and biologically active chromium per tablespoon, has been shown to lower cholesterol. As 200mcg of chromium is the usual amount of chromium supplemented, two tablespoons of Brewer's yeast daily is recommended. Chromium supplementation has shown mixed results on cholesterol levels in human studies, although in 1998, a double blind study using a daily supplement of 500mcg of chromium picolinate reduced total cholesterol by almost 20% over 13 weeks. A more recent trial using 200mcg chromium daily led to significant reductions in serum triglycerides and total cholesterol (Jamilian *et al*, 2018).

Garlic capsules

A meta-analysis of 26 studies by Zeng *et al* (2012) researching the effects of garlic on blood lipids, illustrated a significant reduction in total cholesterol and triglyceride levels. 600 to 900 mg a day of a standardised garlic extract may help lower cholesterol, reduce blood pressure and help to prevent hardening of the arteries. A 2018 trial measured the effects upon arterial stiffness in ninety-two subjects given garlic extract. C-reactive protein (a marker of artery lining function) and LDL were all reduced in the garlic, but not in the placebo group, illustrating that supplementation with garlic extract favourably modifies endothelial biomarkers associated with cardiovascular risk.

Fibre to reduce cholesterol

Beta glucan

Results from a number of double-blind trials have illustrated reductions of approximately 10% less total cholesterol and 8% less LDL cholesterol, with HDL cholesterol often simultaneously increased, in some cases up to 16% higher. Othman *et al* (2011) conducted a meta-analysis of studies conducted during the past 13 years, and found that 3g or more daily of oat β-glucan consumption was associated with reductions of 5% in total cholesterol and 7% in LDL cholesterol.

Glucomannan

Glucomannan is another type of soluble plant fibre. Sood *et al* (2008) conducted a meta-analysis of 14 trials to research the effects of glucomannan, and found statistically significant reductions in total and LDL cholesterol, triglycerides and fasting blood glucose. Effective amounts of glucomannan for lowering blood cholesterol range between 4 to 13 grams daily.

Psyllium husk

Psyllium husk is a type of solube fibre usually used to help alleviate constipation and normalize bowel function. However, it has been shown to have cholesterol-lowering properties, by binding with intestinal cholesterol and increasing its elimination in the faeces. Moreyra *et al* (2005) found that administering 15g of psyllium husk with 10g of simvastatin was as effective as taking 20mg of simvastatin. Taking 5 to 10 grams with meals (1 to 2 teaspoons mixed with water) may help to reduce your cholesterol levels.

Whilst including foods rich in these nutrients will certainly benefit your health, high doses of some substances may be necessary to benefit from some of these therapeutic effects. Effects are individual and will also depend upon the efficacy of the supplement. It is recommended that you consult a qualified professional for help with therapeutic supplementation for any cardiovascular conditions.

Summing Up

To reduce the risk of heart disease:

- Consume foods rich in heart-healthy polyunsaturated and monounsaturated fats (fish, nuts, seeds, vegetable oils, avocado, olives)

- Eat at least five servings of anti-oxidant-rich, potassium-rich fruit and vegetables a day

- Eat two cloves of garlic daily

- Eat beans, oats and inulin-rich asparagus, Jerusalem artichoke and chicory to help reduce circulating cholesterol

- Don't over-eat and keep body fat levels low – especially intra-abdominal visceral fat

- Consume olive oil cold and use at low temperatures for cooking

- Reduce salt intake

- Avoid refined (trans and hydrogenated) fats

- Limit your consumption of sugars and refined carbohydrate foods

- If you do drink alcohol, limit your intake to one – two units daily, and consider swapping to red wine!

Stick to	Stay away from
Fish	Processed fatty foods
Garlic	Refined carbohydrates
Red wine	Too much alcohol
Fruit and vegetables	Salt
Oats, beans and inulin-rich vegetables	Sugar
Olive oil	
Nuts and seeds	

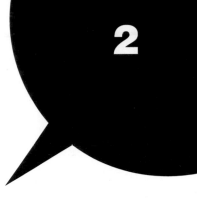

2

Food for better bones and joints

Almost a third of the UK population have some sort of musculoskeletal condition – over 400,000 people in the UK have swollen, stiff and painful joints caused by rheumatoid arthritis (RA), and around 10 mllion have osteoarthritis. The number of arthritis sufferers is increasing: people are living longer and therefore more likely to experience osteoarthritis, and being overweight (also on the increase) exacerbates both of these conditions. Increased use of proton pump inhibitors such as Omeprazole, prescribed to reduce acid reflux, also contribute bone and joint disorders as these medications reduce gastric acid secretion in the stomach, which affects the absorption of several key nutrients, including calcium and iron, both needed for strong bones.

Some experts now consider inflammatory diseases such as arthritis to be a result of systemic inflammatory breakdown – a result of a nutrient-poor diet and/or reduced absorption, and low activity levels. A report comparing the mineral content of fruit, vegetables, meat and milk between 1940 and 2002 showed a significant reduction in key minerals in our food, in some examples up to 70% lower. However, there are a number of dietary and lifestyle factors that either contribute to, or reduce the risk of bone and joint complaints, so you can take control over your skeletal and joint health.

Rheumatoid arthritis

Rheumatoid arthritis is an inflammatory autoimmune condition caused by a combination of genetic and environmental factors. Autoimmune conditions occur when your immune system, which usually fights infection, attacks part of the body. In rheumatoid arthritis the lining of your joints is attacked, causing them to become inflamed, swollen and painful. Initially, the joints of the hands and feet are affected, but any joint may become affected. At present there is no known cure for rheumatoid arthritis, but symptoms can be eased and the progression of the condition can be slowed down.

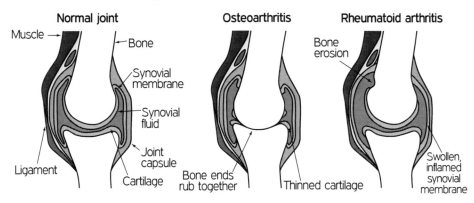

Development of Rheumatoid Arthritis (RA)

Immune cells infiltrate joint fluid and begin to attack bone and cartilage. As the bone becomes eroded, cysts form, and osteoporosis may also occur. Synovial joint fluid, which normally enables easy movement, is displaced by functionless tissue, followed by inflammation and cartilage erosion. Separate bones may even fuse together.

need2know

Risk factors for rheumatoid arthritis

- Women are up to three times more likely to develop rheumatoid arthritis than men

- It occurs most commonly between the ages of 40 and 70, but it can develop at any age

- Being overweight significantly increases the risk of rheumatoid arthritis

- Rheumatoid arthritis in your family increases your risk because certain genes are thought to make some people more susceptible to developing the disease

- It is more common in conjunction with high intakes of coffee or red meat

- Compared to non-smokers, men who smoke are twice as likely to develop RA; women who smoke increase their risk by 1.3 times. Smoking increases the risk by depleting the body of essential anti-oxidants that could otherwise support immune function and help to counteract inflammation.

Arthtritis Research UK, 2018.

It is also less common in people who consume higher amounts of vitamin C, and who consume a moderate amount of alcohol. Although you can't change your age, gender or family history, you can reduce your risk of getting rheumatoid arthritis by not smoking, and making some dietary changes.

'You want to add life to your years as well as years to your life.'

Dietary factors to help combat rheumatoid arthritis

Weight, rheumatoid arthritis and cardiovascular risk

Being overweight (body mass index (BMI) of between 25 and 30) increases your risk of developing rheumatoid arthritis by up to 15%. Being obese (BMI 30 – 35) increases the risk by 21 – 31% compared with those with a healthy weight. Eating less and exercising more (or staying active) will help to maintain a healthy weight and reduce your risk of rheumatoid arthritis. Having rheumatoid arthritis also increases your risk of developing cardiovascular disease and having a stroke or heart attack, so following the dietary guidelines in the previous chapter will help to reduce this risk.

There are a number of other dietary factors that reduce the risk and ameliorate symptoms of rheumatoid arthritis:

- Boost immune function by consuming plenty of anti-oxidants – this can reduce your risk of infection (and therefore reduce your risk of developing rheumatoid arthritis), and help to reduce inflammation in existing cases
- Omit or reduce foods that aggravate symptoms
- Eat foods with anti-inflammatory properties to help reduce inflammation, such as consuming less red meat and eating more fish
- Consider a vegetarian diet.

An anti-inflammatory diet is also recommended for those with osteoarthritis.

Eat foods rich in anti-oxidants

Oxidative stress is elevated in those with RA, which implies that reactive oxygen species (ROS) are possible mediators of tissue damage as they invoke immune responses causing inflammation. Decreasing inflammation and oxidative stress may enhance regeneration of cartilage within the joint, reduce pain, and also reduce cardiovascular risk factors. Research has shown conflicting results with anti-oxidant supplementation, but a diet rich in anti-oxidants should help to reduce inflammation and enhance overall wellbeing. Autoimmune conditions such as rheumatoid arthritis often occur after infection, so eating plenty of anti-oxidant rich foods to boost immune function can help you to stay healthy and not give your immune system an opportunity to turn against you if you don't already suffer with RA.

The anti-oxidants

There are many nutrients in a healthy diet that have anti-oxidant properties, including several vitamins and minerals. The most well known anti-oxidants are vitamins A, C and E. Minerals such as zinc, iron and selenium are also anti-oxidants.

Let's take a look at the foods that are rich sources of these nutrients.

For beta carotene	For vitamin C	For vitamin E
Carrots	Peppers	Nuts
Sweet potato squash	Citrus fruits	Seeds
Apricots	Kiwi	Avocados
Mango	Berries	Vegetable oils
Cantaloupe melon	Green leafy vegetables	Wheat germ
For zinc	**For selenium**	**For iron**
Whole grains	Brazil nuts	Meat
Shellfish	Sunflower seeds	Beans
Dairy foods	Brown rice	Brown rice
Dark cuts of meat	Seafood	Green leafy vegetables
Pumpkin seeds	Eggs	Dried fruit

Although vitamin A is found in dairy foods, it's better to increase your intake of beta carotene, a water-soluble nutrient that is converted into vitamin A as and when it is required, but is water soluble, so won't overdose the body with excess vitamin A. Beta carotene belongs to a group of plant nutrients called carotenes. These are usually found in fruits and vegetables that are red/orange/yellow in colour, but you'll also find them in green leafy vegetables and beetroot.

Vitamin C (ascorbic acid)

Vitamin C scavenges pro-inflammatory reactive oxygen species, supports collagen formation and enhances extracellular matrix protein synthesis. RA patients tend to be vitamin C deficient and require high supplementation doses just to maintain plasma vitamin C at acceptable levels. Very high intravenous doses of vitamin C have been reported to reduce inflammation and ease pain, but these dosages are within medical research trials, so in the absence of conclusive evidence, it is recommended that you eat a diet rich in vitamin C, and consider a 500mg – 1g daily supplement.

Avoiding foods which make your arthritis worse

Some research illustrates increased immune response and flare-ups in rheumatoid arthritis when certain foods are eaten. Karatay *et al* (2004) found that symptoms such as stiffness and pain, and the level of inflammatory markers in the blood all increased when foods that tested positive in an allergic skin prick test were eaten. In further research they again found that symptoms were aggravated when allergenic foods were included in the diet.

Common food allergens

Although allergy tests may illustrate specific foods or substances that you have an allergy to, these tests are sometimes unreliable and usually expensive. Although you may be allergic to, or intolerant of any food, there are some foods that can cause problems much more frequently than others:

- Dairy foods including milk, yoghurt and cheese (particularly cow's milk and cow's milk products)
- Wheat products e.g. bread and pasta
- Gluten (a type of protein found in cereals such as wheat, barley and rye)
- Foods from the Nightshade family (tomatoes, aubergine, peppers, white potatoes)

'Although anyone's health benefits from a rich intake of anti-oxidants, for those suffering with rheumatoid arthritis, an anti-oxidant rich diet is even more therapeutic.'

- Eggs
- Citrus fruits
- Coffee
- Chocolate.

A note on the Nightshade family

This group of foods contains the alkaloids solanine or capsaicin, which can increase joint pain in some individuals. You may not, however, react to all nightshade foods, so treat each one individually. Potatoes that have green spots or have sprouted will have higher levels of solanine. Conversely, capsaicin has anti-inflammatory properties and is used topically to reduce inflammation and pain in arthritis. There are many other foods in the Nightshade family, so it may be worth checking out a complete list of them (see the Help List at the back of this book). Other foods such as blueberries and Goji berries, although not part of the Nightshade family, contain a similar alkaloid, and may affect you if you are susceptible to this component in foods.

How to follow an exclusion diet

If you suspect that some foods are exacerbating your arthritis you might want to exclude them from your diet.

1 The first step is to remove either suspect foods or common allergens from your diet. Ideally, an allergen should be excluded for three weeks to allow all traces to be removed from the body, although you may notice a difference immediately, or within a few days. When trying to identify a food allergen, you can exclude more than one suspect food simultaneously by removing all suspected foods at once, but you must re-introduce each food individually otherwise it is impossible to know which food may be aggravating your symptoms. Once a food is excluded, you should note any change/improvement in symptoms.

2 The second stage is to re-introduce foods back into the diet and monitor your symptoms. If a food appears to cause no symptoms, you can keep it in your diet. If symptoms return or worsen, you then need to decide whether you want to continue eating that food, with the resulting symptoms, or exclude it from your diet.

'Whilst you continue to eat foods which you are knowingly or unknowingly intolerant of, these foods stimulate your immune system to create symptoms such as inflammation, and increase your requirement for anti-oxidants.'

3 During the exclusion diet it's a good idea to keep a food diary to see how certain foods affect your arthritis. Mark each common symptom such as stiffness or pain zero to five so that you can measure the effects of excluding and then re-introducing foods in your diet.

There is an exclusion diet in the Appendices to help get you started.

It is best to consult a nutritionist or dietician before excluding any major food or food group from the diet to avoid creating nutrient deficiencies and to ensure that your diet is balanced. If you are breast feeding, pregnant or taking any medication, you should also consult with your doctor before making any dietary changes. It can be difficult to remove all traces of some substances, as products from milk, eggs and wheat are added to many processed foods. A qualified practitioner will help you to plan an effective exclusion diet that is also healthy and balanced, and not lacking in any nutrients.

An anti-inflammatory diet for rheumatoid and osteoarthritis

Joint inflammation is a key symptom in both types of arthritis, and this is the main symptom of arthritis that may be alleviated through diet.

There are several foods that contain nutrients with anti-inflammatory properties:

- Fish
- Nuts, seeds and their oils
- Onions
- Green leafy vegetables
- Pineapple.

Let's take a look at how these foods can reduce inflammatory conditions, and how to include them in your diet.

Adjusting your fatty acid profile

The types of fats that we eat contribute to our natural anti-inflammatory and pro-inflammatory pathways, and in good health these are balanced. However, an imbalanced intake of fats over a period of time can cause us to be overly 'inflammatory', so the inflammatory symptoms of arthritis may improve with an 'anti-inflammatory diet'. One of the key elements of such a diet is re-balancing the types of fats that you eat.

As the only naturally rich sources of 'anti-inflammatory' omega 3 fatty acids are fish, algae, walnuts and linseeds and their related oils, many people, especially non-fish eaters, struggle to include enough of these essential fats in their diet. Although many foods contain omega 3 and omega 6 fatty acids, very few have a healthy omega 6: omega 3 ratio, so over time it is possible to have an unbalanced fatty acid intake as shown below:

Normal healthy ratio	3:1 (omega 6: omega 3)
Typical western diet ratio	16-20:1 (omega 6: omega 3)

'In patients given an anti-inflammatory diet, the numbers of tender and swollen joints decreased by 14%, and adding fish oil supplements led to a further significant reduction in the numbers of tender and swollen joints'

(Adam *et al*, 2003).

After following such a diet for a number of years, many of us need to adjust our fatty acid ratio in favour of the omega 3 fats to correct an imbalance and reduce inflammatory conditions. As both types of fatty acids affect our inflammatory pathways, if we have too much of one type of fat and not enough of the other, we often experience symptoms such as the inflammation common to arthritis. We need lots of different nutrients to ensure that these pathways are effective, but consuming a correct ratio of essential fatty acids in your diet is a good place to start.

Check the lists below to see if you are eating enough omega 6 and omega 3.

Foods rich in omega 3	Foods rich in omega 6
Oily fish	Margarines
Linseeds (flaxseeds)	Vegetable oils
Walnuts	Nuts and seeds

Most seeds and nuts contain both types of fat, but usually contain more of the omega 6 fats. This table shows the omega 3 and omega 6 fatty acid contents of some nuts, seeds and oils. Remember, to reduce inflammatory symptoms, you need more omega 3 oils and fewer omega 6.

The omega 3 and omega 6 fatty acid content of nuts, seeds and oils

	Omega 3 (g/100g)	Omega 6 (g/100g)
Linseed/linseed oil	51.5	13
Walnut	7	36
Brazil nut	0	23.5
Almonds	0.3	10
Sunflower seeds	0.14	24.6
Sunflower oil	0.27	46.8
Olive oil	0.6	9.9

All figures are for uncooked foods. Source of information: McCance and Widdowson's 'The Composition of Foods Integrated Dataset', 2015.

Omega 3 rich oils

- Olive oil is not particularly rich in omega 3 fats, but contains considerably less omega 6 fats than most other oils

- Rapeseed oil is a rich source of omega 3 fats and also has less than half the amount of omega 6 fats found in other vegetable oils such as sunflower oil

- Linseed oil contains an even lower proportion of omega 6 fats and has the highest amount of omega 3 oils available in a vegetable oil.

Our body fat is made up of the type of fatty acids we commonly eat, so if you have eaten very little fish, linseeds or walnuts over a number of years, your body fat may contain an unbalanced ratio of fatty acids. Whenever you break down your body fat for energy, the fatty acids are released into the blood stream, so don't expect to correct a fatty acid imbalance overnight. If you think this applies to you, avoid foods such as sunflower seeds, which contain more omega 6 fats than omega 3, as this will slow down your efforts to correct your fatty acid imbalance.

Ways to add omega-3 rich linseeds, walnuts and oils to your diet

- Add linseeds and walnuts to cereals, yoghurts, salads and stir fries

- Try bars with added seeds such as the '9 bar' with linseeds

- Just nibble on walnuts
- Cook with olive oil
- Add rapeseed oil, walnut oil, edible linseed oil or olive oil to salads.

Meat versus fish

'The IOWA
Women's
Health
study
in 2004
reported
a link
between
low levels
of vitamin
D and
rheumatoid
arthritis,
giving
an extra
reason to
eat oily
fish rich in
Vitamin D.'

Meats are rich in an omega 6 fatty acid called arachidonic acid, that leads to the formation of inflammatory 2-series prostaglandins and 4-series leukotrienes. Non-steroidal anti-inflammatory drugs used in rheumatoid arthritis work by decreasing the production of 2-series prostaglandins. As arachidonic acid promotes our pro-inflammatory pathways, eating too much meat may promote inflammation, and consumption of red meat has been linked with a higher occurrence of rheumatoid arthritis. If you have consumed more meat than fish over a number of years, you may find it beneficial to swap your ratio around, for example, eating more fish than meat, or even omitting meat from your diet for a while.

Ways to swap pro-inflammatory foods for anti-inflammatory foods

- Swap meat, eggs or cheese for fresh or tinned fish in sandwiches
- Swap cheese on toast to sardines on toast
- Swap omelette or eggs for breakfast to kedgeree or kippers
- Swap roast meats at dinner for salmon or tuna steak
- Use tuna or soya mince in place of mince in pasta dishes.

Long term and consistent intake of fish or fish oil supplements has a protective effect against rheumatoid arthritis. However, vegetarian and vegan diets also seem to convey some benefits, probably due to antioxidant constituents, fibre intake, and by the resultant changes in intestinal flora. In their review of research trials testing the effects of different diets on rheumatoid arthritis, Smedslund *et al* (2010) found that fasting followed by 13 months on a vegetarian eating plan may reduce pain, and following a Mediterranean eating plan for 12 weeks also reduced pain. Outcomes from vegan diets were less conclusive, but all diets induced weight loss, which would reduce systemic inflammation and may be at least one parameter involved in reducing pain.

Other anti-inflammatory foods and spices

Onions

All types of onion contain a phytonutrient called quercetin, which belongs to the flavonoid family. Flavonoids have so many health benefits that they are sometimes referred to as 'Vitamin P'. As well as being anti-inflammatory, onions are also known to be:

- Anti-histamine
- Anti-viral
- Anti-bacterial
- Anti-allergic.

Green leafy vegetables and brassicas

These types of vegetable contain some omega 3 fatty acids and they are also a rich source of anti-oxidant nutrients such as iron, beta carotene and vitamin C, which all support immune function.

Pineapple

Fresh pineapple contains an enzyme called bromelain that has anti-inflammatory properties. Most research on anti-arthritic agents (medications) is tested on rats, as they exhibit the most similar responses to humans. A trial on rats with induced rheumatoid arthritis illustrated that pineapple extract decreased blood levels of inflammatory C-reactive protein and PGE2prostaglandins (Kargutkar and Brijesh, 2016). In 1964, Cohen and Goldman conducted a clinical study, illustrating that bromelain decreased swelling and pain in 72% of rheumatoid arthritis patients.

Spices – Turmeric and ginger

Curcumin (a curcuminoid) is the main active constituent in the spice turmeric. Numerous studies have illustrated its anti-inflammatory properties and it has also been shown to reduce the action of collagenase, the enzyme that breaks down the constituents of cartilage (Zhang *et al*, 2016). However, curcuminoids have poor solubility in chyme and are unstable in the digestive tract pH, so only a small fraction of ingested curcuminoids is absorbed. In addition, curcuminoids undergo rapid metabolism, so they don't stay in circulation in the body for long. Curcuminoid absorption is better when consumed with fats or oils in food, as they are lipophilic (they attach to fats). You should take turmeric

'Shiitake mushrooms contain beta glucan, which enhances immune function. Add to miso soup or sauté with onions, garlic, tofu, bean sprouts and mange tout for a healthy stir fry.'

supplements with meals for the same reason, or choose a supplement that includes a bioavailability enhancer such as micelles, which is designed to enhance its solubility and stability in the gastrointestinal tract.

Ginger is traditionally used as an anti-inflammatory in Chinese and Ayurvedic medicine, and although scientific evidence of ginger's anti-arthritic effects is sparse, it has been shown to share pharmacological properties with non-steroidal anti-inflammatory drugs, suppressing the synthesis of inflammatory compounds, but without any of the side effects.

Oregano and rosemary also have anti-inflammatory properties and should be used frequently in cooking.

How to include more of these foods in your diet

- Add onions and rocket, watercress or spinach to sandwiches, wraps and salads
- Add watercress or rocket to rice and pasta dishes
- Start stir fries, casseroles, stews and soups off with an onion
- Add onion and green leaves to omelettes and savoury souffles
- Add turmeric to stews, curries, chillies, casseroles and stir fries
- Add ginger to desserts or soups
- Drink ginger tea.

There is an anti-inflammatory eating plan in the Appendices.

Osteoarthritis

Osteoarthritis is the most common joint disorder in the UK and is on the rise. This is thought to be due to increased levels of obesity and the fact that we are generally living longer. It is also known as degenerative joint disease because the condition is due to the increased break down of the joints, specifically the cartilage on the ends of the bones that normally stops bones rubbing together. Although there is a gap between the bones, which is filled with lubricating synovial fluid, the cartilage still aids joint movement, and symptoms arise as a result of joint degeneration and the body's attempts to repair the damage. Osteoarthritis usually affects weight-bearing joints such as the hips and knees, though it can occur in the hands and wrists.

Risk factors for osteoarthritis

- Risk of developing osteoarthritis increases with age

- The prevalence of osteoarthritis is generally higher in women than men

- Genetic factors account for 60% of hand and hip osteoarthritis and 40% of knee osteoarthritis

- Prolonged wear and tear or overuse of joints, particularly weight bearing joints – knee arthritis is generally associated with long intervals of kneeling or squatting, hip arthritis is linked with prolonged standing or lifting, and jobs or hobbies requiring manual dexterity increases the risk of arthritis in the hands and wrists

- Uneven weight bearing or unbalanced joint positioning, especially in the hips

- High levels of collagenase (an enzyme that breaks down the collagen that forms cartilage)

- Inflammation from bony outgrowths may cause uneven loading

- Excess weight – people who are overweight are 2.5 times more likely to develop arthritis in the knees, and obesity increases the risk by 4.6 times.

Metabolic syndrome (the combined presence of diabetes, high blood pressure and obesity) is prevalent in 59% of people with osteoarthritis compared to 23% of people without osteoarthritis. Obesity and elevated blood glucose levels both increase inflammation in the body, and the excess weight increases the strain on joints, so the link between these diseases is clear to see.

Dietary adjustments to help with osteoarthritis

An anti-inflammatory eating plan such as the one included in the Appendices, and the anti-inflammatory dietary measures included for rheumatoid arthritis will be helpful in reducing inflammatory symptoms of osteoarthritis. In addition, due to the high prevalence of metabolic syndrome in those with osteoarthritis, and clear links between both obesity and blood glucose dysregulation and this degenerative joint complaint, a diet low in carbohydrates with portion control to induce a healthy weight is also recommended.

Supplements to help rheumatoid and osteoarthritis

Eicosapentanoic acid (EPA), docosahexanoic acid (DHA) and cod liver oil

Cod liver oil is a well-known remedy for joint problems, but although cod liver oil is a fish oil, EPA and DHA fish oil supplements are more commonly prescribed in nutritional therapy. EPA and DHA are derived from the body flesh of fish, usually oily fish such as sardines, mackerel or salmon, whereas cod liver oil takes its oil from the cod liver.

'Essential fatty acids are also thought to play a role in calcium absorption and metabolism in the body, so a fish oil supplement may also benefit osteoporosis.'

- Fish such as cod store much of their fat along with fat-soluble vitamins such as vitamins A and D in the liver, so these vitamins may be present in cod liver oil supplements. Vitamin A is a strong antioxidant that can prevent cell damage by interacting with harmful molecules called free radicals. Vitamin D plays an important role in the production of proteoglycan in cartilage, and also enhances the absorption of calcium, an essential mineral for strong bones. However, although Vitamin A is essential in our diet, high intakes can be detrimental to health, so vitamin A supplementation is safer in the form of beta carotene. Supplements containing fatty acids from fish liver or fish flesh may have additional vitamins such as vitamin A or D added to them anyway.

- As the liver is an organ of detoxification, high levels of contaminants such as mercury or polychlorinated biphenyls (PCBs) may be present in cod liver oil supplements, although these pollutants can occur in any fish oil supplement even if the oils have been extracted from the flesh of the fish rather than the liver.

- It is the anti-inflammatory properties of fish oils that may help to reduce inflammation. Cod liver oil capsules do not contain the same levels of EPA and DHA omega 3 oils, making them less effective than fish oil supplements that may provide more EPA or DHA in a daily dose.

Akbar *et al* (2017) reviewed trials using fish oils on inflammatory conditions. They found that 16 out of 20 trials involving rheumatoid arthritis, and 3 out of 4 trials involving osteoarthritis showed significant improvements. Another systematic review of trials concluded that daily supplementation of 3g – 6g of omega 3 fatty acid had a therapeutic effect upon pain levels (Abdulrazaq *et al*, 2017).

Gamma linoleic acid (GLA) (from Evening Primrose, Starflower or Borage oil)

A systematic review including seven different research trials using GLA concluded that there is moderate evidence of this oil reducing symptoms in rheumatoid arthritis (Cameron, Gagnier and Chrubasik, 2011). Various amounts of GLA, between 1g to 3g were used daily, sometimes in conjunction with fish oils.

Vitamin D for RA

Vitamin D levels are lower in those with rheumatoid arthritis, and vitamin D levels also correlate inversely with RA activity – the lower the vitamin D status, the worse the RA condition appears to be. A 2016 meta-analysis of 15 studies concluded that the vitamin D level is associated with both susceptibility to RA and RA activity (Lee and Bae, 2016). In addition, suboptimal vitamin D status is now acknowledged as an independent predictor of cardiovascular disease and osteoporosis (both conditions that occur more frequently in those with RA). Milk and dairy alternative milks, breakfast cereals, and some orange juices are fortified with vitamin D, and it is naturally found in egg yolks, salmon, tuna, and sardines.

However, as we make most of our vitamin D in the skin when we come into contact with sunshine, vitamin D levels can be significantly lower through winter and in those spending more time indoors or using sunscreen. Therefore, a vitamin D supplement can be helpful. Adults up to age 70 should take 600 IU of vitamin D per day, 800 IU daily for those over 70.

Vitamin K(2) for RA

Vitamin K is known to improve bone density in osteoporosis, and it appears that it can improve rheumatoid arthritis too. Ebina *et al* (2013) found significantly lower levels of C-reactive protein, an inflammatory marker, in the blood plasma of those who had supplemented with K2. A separate 2015 clinical study showed reduced levels of several markers for RA activity, suggesting that vitamin K2 improves disease activity in RA patients (Abdel-Rahman *et al*, 2015).

Vitamin E for RA

People with RA seem to suffer with impaired anti-oxidant systems, making them more susceptible to free radical damage. Vitamin E is an important anti-oxidant that protects joints against oxidative damage. Low vitamin E levels in the joint fluid of people with

RA have been reported, and Aryaelan *et al* (2011) found plasma concentration of anti-oxidants including vitamin E were lower than in controls. In one double-blind trial, 1,800 IU per day of vitamin E reduced pain from RA. Two other double-blind trials (using similar amounts of vitamin E) reported that vitamin E had the same effectiveness in reducing symptoms of RA as anti-inflammatory drugs. In other double-blind trials, 600 IU of vitamin E taken twice daily was significantly more effective than placebo in reducing pain. However, taking 600IU every other day was found to have no significant effect upon reducing the risk of developing rheumatoid arthritis (Karlson *et al*, 2008).

Folic acid for RA

Some drugs used for rheumatoid arthritis such as methotrexate (Rheumatrex, Trexall) and sulfasalazine (Azulfidine) interfere with how the body uses folic acid, so it is recommended that if you take these drugs, you might benefit from a folic acid supplement containing at least 400mcg daily. Some experts recommend 1mg of folic acid every day or 5mg once a week. You can find 400mcg of folate in a good multi-vitamin/mineral supplement.

Curcumin for OA and RA

A review on several studies measuring the effectiveness of curcumin concluded that the trials provided scientific evidence to support the efficacy of turmeric extract (about 1000mg/day) in the treatment of arthritis (Daily *et al*, 2016).

Glucosamine and chondroitin for OA

Cartilage is largely made up of molecular structures called glycosaminoglycans, made from carbohydrate and protein foods. Osteoarthritis is partly due to an exaggerated break down of cartilage, but simply eating more of the foods that we make cartilage from won't have an effect – your body will just use the additional foods for other purposes, or lay any excess down as body fat, which exacerbates the condition. If it is unlikely that your diet is lacking in protein or carbohydrate, the cartilage formation disruption is enzyme-related.

Glucosamine and chondroitin are amongst the most common types of supplement taken for osteoarthritis. These supplements contain the nutrients we use to form cartilage in the body. Glucosamine is an amino sugar that the body produces and distributes in cartilage and other connective tissue, forming proteoglycans; chondroitin sulphate is a complex carbohydrate that helps cartilage retain water. Some arthritis sufferers report positive results after taking these supplements, however, in a large scale trial in the US involving

1583 people with osteoarthritis called the Glucosamine/chondroitin Arthritis Intervention Trial (GAIT), the effects of glucosamine hydrochloride and chondroitin sulphate were tested over 24 weeks, and only those with moderate to severe pain experienced pain relief taking glucosamine combined with chondroitin sulphate. Extended research to study improvements in knee cartilage over two years with 581 participants showed no reduction in the loss of knee cartilage. Some researchers suggest that effects of this supplement depend upon the enzymic activity rate on cartilage breakdown.

Methyl sulphonyl methane

Methyl sulphonyl methane (MSM) is a sulphur supplement, and is often used in conjunction with chondroitin or glucosamine. It seems to increase the effectiveness of these supplements and also help to ease pain. In a systematic review of published research on foods and supplements affecting osteoarthritis, Ameye and Chee (2008) found good evidence for avocado and soybean extracts, and moderate evidence that methyl sulphonyl methane provides symptom relief to osteoarthritic patients.

Cherry extract for OA

It is possible that cherry extract may help reduce symptoms of osteoarthritis – in one study, patients who consumed two 8-ounce bottles of tart cherry juice daily for 6 weeks experienced a significant improvement in pain, stiffness and physical function, and showed a marked decrease in C-reactive protein (CRP), a marker of inflammation. Each bottle of juice contained the equivalent of about 45 cherries. A 2007 pilot study also reported improved pain and function after participants took one cherry capsule a day for eight weeks.

Bromelain for OA

Treatment with 500mg of bromelain for 3-4 weeks has been found to be as effective for treatment of knee osteoarthritis as 100mg diclofenac.

Calcium for arthritis and osteoporosis

Corticosteroids taken for arthritis can reduce the absorption of calcium from your diet, which can increase the risk of osteoporosis and other health conditions. If you take corticosteroids it is recommended that adults younger than 50 take 1000 mg (1g) of calcium daily, and women over 50/men over 70 take 1200mg. However, some evidence shows no benefit regarding osteoporosis from supplementing with additional calcium alone, or even calcium with vitamin D, so finding a natural anti-inflammatory alternative to corticosteroids may be a better option to protect bone health.

If you are taking any medication you should always check with your doctor before taking any supplements. It is also recommended that you consult a qualified nutritional practitioner to help you adjust your diet and decide upon the right supplementation.

Osteoporosis

'Falls are a major cause of disability and the leading cause of mortality due to injury in people aged over 75 in the UK.'
National Osteoporosis Society.

Over 3 million people in the UK have osteoporosis. In osteoporosis the bones are more porous due to a lack of calcium phosphate. This makes them more liable to fracture easily, although there are often no symptoms until a fracture occurs. Menopausal women can experience a loss of 5 – 10% bone density each year due to reducing oestrogen levels, and up to 40% of women may suffer with osteoporosis by age 80, although the condition can be delayed or even reduced through diet and exercise. Both men and women usually suffer with some bone density loss as we age. The most effective prevention is to maximise bone mineral density whilst bone tissue is still forming (before age 35) with weight bearing exercise and a balanced diet.

Risk factors for osteoporosis

- Lack of regular weight bearing exercise or long periods of immobility

- Very low body weight

- Age, race and gender (more common as we age, in those of black afro-Caribbean origin, and in post-menopausal women)

- Reduced levels of hormones such as oestrogen or testosterone which promote bone building

- Other medical conditions such as rheumatoid arthritis, hyperthyroidism or parathyroid disease

- Smoking depletes essential nutrients that would have otherwise contributed to healthy bone tissue – the risk of fractures can be increased by up to 15% with this unhealthy habit

- Long term use of corticosteroids, contraceptive pills, anti-convulsants, anti-depressants, blood coagulants and thyroid medications, as all of these affect nutrient absorption and/or increase nutrient loss

- Chronic stress – sustained high levels of the stress hormone cortisol increases inflammation and bone mineral loss

- Drinking more than two cups of coffee daily

- Drinking more than two units of alcohol a day

- Drinking fizzy drinks that contain phosphoric acid can increase the risk of fractures

- Excessive salt intake

- Excessive protein intake

- Lack of essential nutrients in the diet, or malabsorption of nutrients (which means you are eating enough but just not absorbing enough of the nutrients into your body) – malabsorption is likely in those with conditions such as coeliac disease or Crohn's disease.

Use it or lose it!

We build bone tissue as required, so the more regularly we place a certain amount of strain on the bones, the more bone tissue is laid down to make the skeletal structure stronger. With a sedentary lifestyle not even involving much walking around, bone tissue will reduce and weaken, sometimes leading to osteoporosis. Although it is advisable to strengthen the bones before the age of approximately 35, it's never too late to start a weight bearing exercise regime. Weight bearing exercise is activity that requires the body, or parts of the body to take the strain of your body weight, or work against the resistance of weights, resistance bands or water. Here are some examples of weight bearing exercise – ideally you need to do one of these at least four to five times weekly.

- Walking and hiking

- Jogging or running

- Stair climbing

- Gym machines such as the cross trainer or stepper

- Yoga or pilates

- Tai Chi or other martial arts

- Weight training
- Fitness or dance classes.

However, too much exercise or insufficient food intake leading to a low, unhealthy body weight will contribute to osteoporosis as the body begins to take essential nutrients from the bones, which weakens them.

How age and gender affects our bones

Although we can affect how much bone tissue is laid down with regular exercise, as we age, our hormone levels alter, and this also affects our bones. Some hormones (natural anabolic hormones such as oestrogen and testosterone) promote the lay down of tissues such as bone, so when levels of these hormones reduce, less bone tissue is formed. This is why reducing amounts of oestrogen during and after the menopause increase the risk of osteoporosis.

'Although more research is needed, it appears that phytoestrogens can enhance the lay down of bone tissue.'

Reduced oestrogen levels can be partially offset by replacing the natural oestrogens with plant oestrogens called phytoestrogens. These nutrients affect our cells in more subtle, but similar ways to natural oestrogen. Studies have looked at the low rates of osteoporosis (and breast cancer) in Japanese women who traditionally consume high levels of phytoestrogens in their diet (around 40mg/day), compared to the higher rates of these diseases in the UK, where we eat fewer phytoestrogen-rich foods (around 3mg/day), and research suggests that we may benefit from eating more phytoestrogenic foods.

Foods rich in phytoestrogens

- Soya products such as soya beans, soya milk, soya yoghurt and tofu
- Chick peas, lentils and mung beans
- Fruits such as apples, plums and cherries
- Peppers, yams, tomatoes, olives, carrots, fennel, potatoes and aubergine.

How to add phytoestrogen rich foods to your diet

- Add soy yoghurt, plums, cherries and apples to breakfast
- Replace dairy milk with soya milk
- Snack on plums, cherries, apples, olives, peppers and carrots

- Add tofu to stir fries
- Fill up on lentil soup
- Add chick peas to salads, curries and stir fries
- Snack on hummus (made with chick peas)
- Use frozen soya beans as a vegetable staple.

How your diet affects your bones

As osteoporosis is a condition identified by porous bones, any dietary factors that may increase mineral loss from the bones will contribute to this condition. There are several dietary habits that can contribute to bone loss:

- Coffee consumption
- Alcohol consumption
- Fizzy drinks
- Too much salt
- High protein diets
- Not enough bone-building nutrients.

Coffee consumption

Coffee has a diuretic effect upon the body – it makes us produce more urine. Whilst this is a natural mechanism, whenever we form urine, essential minerals such as calcium and magnesium may be excreted. Without a diuretic effect, more of these minerals remain in the blood stream and are available to be laid down as bone tissue, but if lost in urine production, calcium in particular is then drawn out of the bones to replenish the calcium lost from the bloodstream. Tea does not appear to have the same effect as coffee.

'Drinking approximately eight cups of coffee daily can increase mineral loss in the urine.'

How your alcoholic tipple affects your bones

Alcohol intake has been linked with decreased bone density, and therefore higher risk of osteoporosis. There appears to be no detrimental effect when alcohol intake is low; in fact some studies have shown better bone density in those that drink sparingly than in abstainers. However, drinking more than one drink daily affects the intake, absorption and metabolism of nutrients such as zinc, and leads to poor bone structure.

Fizzy drinks 'dissolve' bone tissue

'A linear relationship exists between bone density and alcohol consumption. Compared with abstainers and heavier drinkers, those who consume 0.5 to 1 drink per day have a lower risk of hip fracture.'

(Berg *et al*, 2008).

Calcium phosphate is the main component of bone tissue, but as with all things in life, too much of a good thing isn't always good for us! Calcium and phosphate levels are closely controlled in the body, and excess minerals excreted out of the body in urine. If there is too much phosphorus in the blood, excess is passed out in urine, but calcium tends to be excreted with it, potentially leading to a calcium deficiency. Phosphate is present in many foods, and added to fizzy drinks (as phosphoric acid) and processed foods – the best way to reduce your phosphorus intake is to replace fizzy drinks with milk, juice, herbal tea or water.

Salt intake

The amount of salt (sodium chloride) in our diet affects the amount of water we retain in our blood stream – high sodium levels lead to elevated blood pressure. Fluid and salt levels are closely controlled through urine formation in the kidneys, so if there is too much sodium in the blood stream, this can lead to higher calcium and magnesium losses in the urine, which reduces availability of these minerals for bone formation.

How much salt should I eat?

The current recommendation is to not exceed 6g of salt a day, but you should preferably aim for less. At present, the average intake in the UK is approximately 9g per day. One way to offset the effects of excess sodium and reduce calcium loss in urine is to consume plenty of potassium, found in fruits and vegetables. For more tips on how to reduce your salt intake, refer back to Chapter 1 'Food for a healthy heart'.

Eat adequate but not excessive amounts of protein

The increased risk of muscle loss and osteoporosis as we age can be attenuated through healthy lifestyle changes, which include adequate dietary protein, alongside regular physical activity. Protein intake and exercise are the main anabolic stimuli for muscle synthesis, and adequate protein intake and resistance exercise contribute to bone density and strength. The European Society for Clinical and Economic Aspects of Osteoporosis and Osteoarthritis (ESCEO) recommends optimal dietary protein intake of 1.0-1.2g per kg bodyweight daily, with at least 20-25g of high-quality protein at each main meal.

However, although we require protein to make strong bones, too much protein in the diet can result in loss of calcium and magnesium salts being leached out of the bone as these minerals are used to offset the resulting acidity created by excess protein, particularly on a high fat, low carbohydrate diet where ketosis occurs. One of the ways we re-balance this is by using calcium and magnesium salts to buffer (neutralize) the acidic substances in the blood, and the largest reservoir of these minerals is in the bone. Considering the detrimental metabolic and inflammatory effects of excess carbohydrate in the diet, the ESCEO recommendations for protein intake are sound, if protein intake provides approximately 20% of dietary calorie intake.

Nutrients for healthy bones

In addition to protein, bone tissue is mostly made up of calcium, phosphorus and magnesium, but several vitamins and minerals are required for the healthy manufacture and sustenance of bone. These nutrients and the foods they are found in are listed below.

Calcium

Calcium is essential for bone formation. It is found in dairy products, dark green leafy and cruciferous vegetables, seeds, beans and tinned sardines. However, despite this mineral being prescribed by doctors when osteoporosis is diagnosed, there is no substantial evidence of reductions in bone loss or fractures as a result of supplementing with calcium. A systematic review carried out by Bolland *et al* in 2015 concluded that most studies reported no association between dietary calcium intake and fracture, and that there was bias toward calcium supplements in the research showing favorable results (reduced risk of fractures) with calcium supplementation. In randomised controlled trials at lowest risk of bias, there was no effect on risk of fractures.

After a review of the evidence, the United States Preventive Services Task Force (USPSTF) concluded that supplementation of calcium and vitamin D for the primary prevention of fractures should not be recommended (2015). In addition, there are an increasing number of studies reporting increased risk of cardiovascular disease following calcium supplementation, although dietary calcium intake shows no increased risk. From this evidence, it is recommended that a rich dietary intake of calcium and

'Bias towards calcium supplementation has been shown in previous studies on the benefits of supplementing with calcium to reduce the risk of osteoporosis or fractures.'

other nutrients needed for healthy bones is consumed, rather than high dose calcium supplements. A better option (in conjunction with a healthy diet), is a multi-nutrient containing magnesium, zinc, iron, selenium, copper, manganese, silicon, boron, and vitamins D and K, which may contain a small amount of calcium.

Magnesium

'If you are housebound or cover your skin for health or religious reasons you may benefit from a vitamin D supplement. Many individuals would benefit from taking 600IU throughout the year, increasing to 1000IU in Winter.'

Deficiency of this mineral increases your risk of osteoporosis as it works in conjunction with calcium and helps vitamin D synthesis. It is found in leafy vegetables, cauliflower, seeds, nuts, pulses and dairy produce.

Vitamin D

Viamin D is needed for calcium and phosphorus absorption and metabolism; we make approximately 90% of our vitamin D requirements in the skin in response to sun exposure. As we make most of our vitamin D in the summer, it's essential that we store enough to get us through winter, although we can still make some vitamin D on cloudy days. Sun block will prevent vitamin D production, but it is thought that only 15 to 20 minutes sun exposure to the arms and face three to four times weekly is required to make enough vitamin D for the year. However, vitamin D deficiency seems to be increasing, and the Scientific Advisory Committee on Nutrition (SACN) recommend supplementation throughout the year in the UK (SACN, 2016). Vitamin D is also found in oily fish, fortified margarines and cereals.

Vitamin E

Tocotrienols (a type of vitamin E) have been found to increase bone density, particularly during menopause. This vitamin quences free radicals, reducing oxidative stress and inflammation. It also reduces osteoclast actiivty – osteoclasts are cells that break down bone tissue, usually working in balance with osteoblasts, cells that build bone tissue (Johnson et al, 2016).

Sulphur

Sulphur is required to build bone, cartilage and connective tissues, and can enhance calcium absorption. It is found in eggs, garlic, onions, and asparagus.

Zinc

This mineral helps to regulate bone tissue growth, and is found in whole grains, meat, pumpkin seeds, liver, wheat germ, Brazil and pecan nuts, shellfish and oysters.

Vitamin C

Vitamin C aids collagen formation to maintain bone strength, and also enhances iron absorption. It is found in berries, peppers, tomatoes, potatoes, dark green leafy vegetables and citrus fruit.

Vitamin K

Vitamin K helps to form proteins used in building bone and promotes bone healing. Recent research shows that K2 (menaquinone-7), a particular type of vitamin K, reduces bone loss and promotes bone strength (Rønn *et al*, 2016). K2 has greater bioavailability than other types of vitamin K, so look for this type of vitamin K in supplements. People with osteoporosis often have low levels of vitamin K, suggesting it may have preventative qualities. Vitamin K is found in green leafy vegetables, broccoli, cauliflower and soya beans.

Vitamin B12

This vitamin is required for methylation pathways in the human body, some of which are involved in building bone tissue. Many medications such as Metformin, proton pump inhibitors (for acid reflux) and diuretics used to reduce blood pressure promote B12 loss in the urine. B12 rich foods include eggs, fish, tofu, dairy foods and meat.

Copper

Nearly 20% of the body's copper is in the bones where it helps to build bone tissue. This mineral is found in nuts and seeds, mushrooms, crab and fruit.

Manganese

A lack of manganese can contribute to osteoporosis. It is present in leafy vegetables, nuts, seeds, meat, pulses and whole grains.

Silicon

This mineral keeps bones and connective tissues healthy, and may increase bone density. You can find silicon in oats, barley and rice.

Boron

Boron has been shown to reduce urinary calcium excretion and increase oestrogen levels. It is found in nuts, dairy products, apples, pears, grapes and green leafy vegetables.

With a long list of nutrients like this, it's clear you need to eat a healthy balanced diet for good bone health.

Poor nutrient absorption

Although some foods are rich in calcium, they also contain substances such as phytates or oxalates which bind to calcium and hinder its absorption. This isn't a problem as long as all of your calcium isn't in foods that contain lots of phytates or oxalates – underlining the importance of a varied diet. Oxalic acid is high in spinach and rhubarb, so although these foods contain lots of calcium, most of it is unavailable as the oxalic acid connects to it and stops it being absorbed into the body. Phytic acid is found in bran and the outside of whole grains, so eating these foods at the same time as calcium-rich foods might reduce the amount of calcium you absorb. These foods are still a healthy addition to your diet, but just make sure that you also eat foods such as tinned fish with bones, enriched soya products, other green leafy vegetables or dairy products to ensure adequate calcium intake.

Supplements for osteoporosis

Doctors generally recommend supplementation of 1g of calcium and 400IU of vitamin D daily for those diagnosed with osteoporosis, though this may be different depending on the severity of bone porosity. However, as discussed earlier on, increasing evidence shows no benefit from supplementing with additional calcium, or even calcium with vitamin D, and it may even increase the risk of cardiovascular disease. It seems that the body needs the wider range of nutrients found within bone tissue to create healthy bone.

Gout

Gout affects approximately 1 in 40 people in the UK. It is said to be the most painful form of arthritis, and the amount of people with gout is increasing. In 2012, a 63.9% increase since 1997 was reported – this increase is likely to be linked with increased levels of obesity and insulin resistance syndrome. One of the causes of these metabolic diseases is the increased intake of fructose in additives such as high-fructose corn syrup, and possibly fad diets such as juicing. Fructose leads to the production of uric acid.

Gout is caused as a result of purine degradation – although most uric acid is endogenous (produced in the body), eating foods rich in purines contributes to the amount of uric acid produced from the purines. Uric acid or urate salts are normally carried by the blood and flushed out through the kidneys. Gout symptoms are caused by high levels of urate salts in the blood stream that have formed into crystals in the joints. It is these crystals that cause gout pain and joint inflammation. Symptoms include intensely painful, red, hot and swollen joints, and it most often affects the big toe, although larger joints such as the knee can be affected.

Risk factors for gout

- Men experience more gout than women
- Genetics may play a role in increasing your risk
- Being overweight, especially carrying excess weight around the middle
- Drinking excessive amounts of alcohol
- Eating high purine foods such as seafood, red meat and offal
- High fructose intake
- High cholesterol levels
- Hypertension and/or taking diuretics
- Diabetes
- Chronic kidney disease.

What to eat and drink to reduce the risk of gout

There is a strong association of the insulin resistance syndrome (abdominal obesity, dyslipidaemia, hypertension, raised serum insulin levels and glucose intolerance) with high uric acid levels, so it makes sense to maintain a healthy weight, reduce sugar intake, and moderate carbohydrate intake. Alcohol intake is also linked to gout, so reducing your intake of alcohol (7 calories per gram) will contribute to weight loss and reduce the risk of gout attacks. It is also important to drink plenty of water (aim for 2 litres a day) as this will help to eliminate uric acid out of the body via the kidneys.

Low-fat dairy products, whole grains, nuts and legumes, and less sugary fruits, coffee and vitamin C supplements decrease the risk of gout, whereas red meat, shellfish, some types of fish, fructose-containing drinks and alcohol increase the risk (Torralba *et al*, 2012). Purine-rich vegetables such as asparagus and spinach do not appear to increase gout. Dairy foods like milk, cheese and yogurt help to increase the excretion of uric acid in the body due to a substance in milk called orotic acid – this helps uric acid to be removed by the kidneys (Dalbeth and Palmano, 2011). Some research suggests that drinking coffee in moderation may be associated with a reduced risk of gout.

Cherries or cherry extract may help prevent episodes of gout. Cherries contain proanthocyanidins that have anti-inflammatory properties, and they may also increase uric acid excretion. Drinking tart cherry juice twice a day has been found to temporarily lower the blood uric acid levels for up to eight hours after consumption. One study (Zhang *et al*, 2012) followed 633 patients with gout for a year. It was observed that cherry consumption was associated with a 32% lower risk of acute gout. This increased to 45% if cherry extract was consumed, and gout attacks were 75% lower in those also taking allopurinol as well as cherry extract. Allopurinol alone reduced the risk by 53%.

Foods to avoid

- Offal (for example kidneys or liver) because of high purine content
- Limit consumption of red meat
- Reduce shellfish and some fish (particularly anchovies, tuna and sardines)
- Limit alcohol to no more than 14 units a week, and have several alcohol-free days – alcohol increases the level of uric acid in the blood
- Limit sugary and fizzy drinks as the fructose content in these can increase uric acid levels
- Limit fruit juices as these also increase uric acid levels
- Limit fruits high in fructose (apples, watermelon, mango, pears, dates, raisins).

Supplements for gout

Cherry extract

In an Internet survey, those taking cherry extract supplements or juice had significantly fewer gout flare ups and tended to take less gout medication. Early findings demonstrated that consumption of fresh or canned cherries prevented attacks of arthritis and restored the plasma uric acid concentrations to normal levels in 12 patients (Blau, 1950). Jacob *et al* (2003) investigated the acute effects of ingesting a bolus of

45 sweet cherries in 10 young healthy women. They found that cherry consumption decreased inflammatory markers in the blood, and plasma uric acid concentration was significantly reduced 5 hours after consuming the cherries. In a recent case-crossover study with 633 gout patients, consumption of fresh cherries or cherry extract over a 2-day period was associated with a 35% lower risk of gout attacks compared with no intake of cherries (Zhang *et al*, 2012).

Vitamin C

Higher vitamin C intake is independently associated with a lower risk of gout, and it appears that the risk and prevalence reduces as vitamin C intake increases, up to 1500mg daily (Choi *et al*, 2009). A review of 13 randomised controlled trials concluded that Vitamin C supplementation (average dose 500mg daily) reduced blood uric acid levels (Juraschek *et al*, 2011).

Summing Up

To help reduce the risk and/or occurrence of arthritis

- Maintain a healthy weight and limit intake of sugar and refined carbohydrates
- Include anti-inflammatory foods such as fish, walnuts, linseeds, onions and green leafy vegetables in your diet
- Maintain a healthy fatty acid balance by eating less meat and more fish
- Consider an exclusion diet to avoid foods you may be intolerant of, or foods which may be causing a flare up
- Eat an anti-oxidant rich diet to combat inflammation and support immune function
- Use anti-inflammatory spices such as turmeric and ginger
- Supplement with various nutrients found to help reduce symptoms.

To help avoid or combat osteoporosis

- Base meals on bone building nutrients from nuts, seeds, beans and pulses, fruit and vegetables, fish and soya or dairy produce
- Limit coffee, fizzy drinks and alcohol
- Cut down on salt
- Don't smoke
- Menopausal women should consider phytoestrogen-rich foods or supplements
- Stay active with weight bearing exercise

For gout

- Maintain a healthy weight and avoid gaining weight around the middle
- Reduce and limit alcohol intake
- Limit your consumption of purine-rich animal proteins and seafood
- Reduce sugar and fructose intake
- Consider using cherry juice or a cherry extract supplement
- Take a vitamin C supplement.

3

Sweet but deadly

Many of us live on a blood sugar roller coaster, going from one quick fix to the next, with energy surges fueled by coffee and refined carbohydrate snacks alternating with energy slumps. Sound familiar? However, although our body has natural mechanisms to control blood sugar levels, a poor diet that consistently causes blood glucose or insulin extremes is detrimental to good health, and metabolic imbalances linked with insulin secretion are now being named as a key cause of obesity and cardiovascular disease, as well as diabetes.

One of the reasons for this is that high glucose levels created by some foods result in a substantial insulin release to reduce blood glucose, but in some this results in low glucose levels again, and a further need for caffeine, sugar or quick release carbohydrates. This can create blood sugar highs and lows throughout the day, increasing your need for sugar and stimulants, which in turn tends to lower your intake of wholesome, nutritious foods, increases overall calorie intake, and escalates insulin secretion.

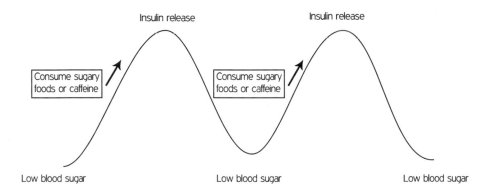

Often, when we have the urge to consume something sweet, these foods also contain high levels of fat or calories. Foods such as sweets, biscuits, doughnuts, chocolate and pastries are commonly used to elevate blood sugar levels, and when considering food intake for the day, you are likely to think you have eaten very little as these 'snacks' are not considered as meals. Calorie intake is often underestimated, leading to weight gain and increasing the risk of diabetes and heart disease. A further problem associated with quick fix carbohydrates is that they are unlikely to be rich sources of vitamins and minerals, so your diet may be lacking in vital nutrients needed for health and energy.

What are carbohydrates?

Although foods are classed as carbohydrates, proteins and fats, most foods are a combination of more than one nutrient, although it is the carbohydrate-rich foods that are associated with affecting our blood sugar levels the most. Carbohydrate foods contain sugars, starch and fibre. A sugar is a simple molecule that is absorbed quickly into the blood stream. Glucose is one of these sugars, and it is glucose that we use for energy. Fibre is made up of chains of sugars that cannot be digested in the human body as we don't possess the digestive enzymes to break them down, although our gut bacteria do partially break down fibre, releasing short chain fatty acids and gases in the colon. Starches are made up of sugar molecules joined together to make larger molecules called polysaccharides (complex carbohydrates) – these tend to take longer to be broken down, digested and absorbed into the blood stream, so polysaccharides can give us a more sustained release of energy, rather than creating the quick surge of energy that foods high in glucose provide. However, some processed complex carbohydrates such as white bread can be digested very quickly and significantly elevate blood glucose levels. It should also be noted that polysaccharides (starches) obviously contain many sugar molecules, and therefore can make a significant contribution to our glycaemic load.

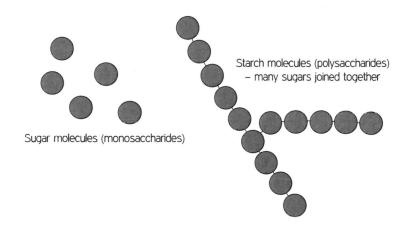

Starch molecules (polysaccharides) – many sugars joined together

Sugar molecules (monosaccharides)

Glucose, a simple sugar, requires no digestion, and is absorbed quickly, raising blood glucose levels. Although other monosaccharides (sugars) such as fructose (found in fruits) or galactose (found in milk products) are also absorbed quickly, they do not have the same immediate effect upon our blood glucose levels, although they are turned into glucose at a later stage, so they too do impact on our overall glucose load.

Foods containing sugars

Sugar
Honey
Syrups
Jams and marmalade
Fruit

Foods rich in non-starch polysaccharides (fibre)

Vegetables (including salad vegetables)
Fruit
Whole grains
Beans and lentils

Carbohydrate-rich foods containing more starchy polysaccharides

Potatoes
Rice
Beans and pulses
Breakfast cereals
Bread
Pasta

Glycaemic Index (GI)

'Riper fruits and vegetables will have a higher GI – a ripe banana contains more sugars than a starchy green banana.'

The Glycaemic Index (GI) is a scale of 1 – 100 indicating how quickly the glucose in foods is absorbed into the blood stream – a low GI will mean the food has low glucose content or contains mostly slow release starches. A high GI score indicates a food that will increase blood glucose levels more quickly. You can choose to eat certain foods based upon their GI to provide you with a more sustained energy release or a quick burst of energy.

Different food brands, cooking methods and even the stage of ripeness alter the GI of foods, but the table below illustrates the average GI of many common foods.

Food	GI	Food	GI
Rice cakes	77	Rye crispbread	63
Easy cook white rice	87	Brown rice	55
White baguette	95	Pumpernickel bread	50
Gluten free bread	90	Oat cakes	54
White bread	70	Rye bread	51
Cous cous	65	Chick peas	28
Puffed wheat	80	Porridge	49
Parsnips	97	Cauliflower	0
Rice pudding	81	Fruit yoghurt	33
Watermelon	72	Grapefruit	25
Pineapple	59	Cherries	22
Chocolate ice cream	68	Strawberry mousse	32
Fizzy orange drink	68	Apple juice	40

Glycaemic Load (GL)

The glycaemic load of a food gives a value according to the effect that a normal portion of the food or drink will have on blood sugar levels. It relates to the type of carbohydrate in a food (the GI) and how much carbohydrate a typical portion contains, and can be calculated as follows:

$$\frac{\text{Glycaemic Index (GI) x the weight (g) of carbohydrate to be eaten}}{100}$$

If you check the carbohydrate grams (g) on a food label, the higher the grams per portion, the higher the GL. If a food has a high GI as well, it will give you a quicker release of energy because the carbohydrates are sugars and more readily absorbed. Although glycaemic index indicates whether a food or drink contains a high proportion of glucose in relation to other sugars, not all high GI foods contain large amounts of glucose. For example, watermelon has a reasonably high GI as most of the sugars are glucose. However, it doesn't have a high glycaemic load as so much of it is water; a typical portion contains only 14g of carbohydrate, in comparison to 40g in a 250ml bottle of Lucozade.

A poor diet and uncontrolled blood glucose levels can contribute to metabolic diseases such as diabetes. Type 2 diabetes is predominantly caused by eating too many carbohydrates, and/or consuming too many calories.

How do we control blood glucose levels?

Whenever we consume carbohydrates or proteins, we produce the hormone insulin that stimulates cellular uptake of amino acids (from protein) and glucose from carbohydrates. Insulin reduces the level of glucose in our bloodstream in a number of ways:

1 It increases the amount of glucose that goes into the cells

2 It increases the conversion of glucose into glycogen (its storage form in the liver and muscles), although the amount we can store is limited to approximately 1600-1700 kcals)

3 It decreases fat breakdown for energy so that we can utilize excess glucose instead

4 It stimulates the conversion of excess glucose into fat.

High levels of insulin are linked to conditions such as obesity, diabetes and heart disease, so although sugary or high GI foods may seem relatively low in calories in comparison to fats, regularly eating these foods is not a good idea for your waistline or your health. It is also less well known that animal proteins also stimulate insulin release with the same effects upon fat metabolism. A focus upon calories and condoning high carbohydrate intake over natural fats in weight loss diets has been a fundamental error in many popular diets supported by slimming clubs, and even some health organizations.

Pre-diabetes

The NHS estimates that one in three adults in the UK have pre-diabetes, which makes them up to 15 times more likely to develop Type 2 diabetes. Symptoms of pre-diabetes are high blood glucose levels and being overweight. The changes that lead to diabetes such as decreased sensitivity to insulin (which means that blood glucose levels remain high) begin several years before symptoms become apparent. With such a high prevalence of blood sugar dysfunction and insulin resistance syndrome in the UK, even if you haven't got diabetes, it's worth making lifestyle changes to ensure that blood sugar regulation stays healthy.

Diabetes Mellitus

More people than ever have diabetes, and due to rising levels of obesity, prevalence of this metabolic disease is still increasing worldwide. According to Diabetes UK there are 4.6 million people with diabetes in the UK, and 12.3 million are at risk, with pre-diabetic conditions such as insulin resistance and metabolic syndrome. Diabetes is diagnosed with an average fasting blood glucose level of 7mmol/l and/or a random plasma glucose concentration of over 11 mmol/l. Fasting blood glucose levels of $\geq$ 6.1mmol/l are an indication of impaired blood sugar regulation and defects in insulin metabolism.

Diabetes mellitus is a group of metabolic diseases characterized by high blood glucose (blood sugar) levels due to defects in insulin secretion or action. Diabetes mellitus means 'sweet urine', so named as high blood glucose levels result in excess glucose being excreted in the urine. Although the term 'diabetes' is commonly used as an umbrella term, there are several different types of diabetes, although Type 1 and Type 2 are the most common. Additional information on other types of diabetes can be found at **www.diabetes.co.uk**.

Risk factors for diabetes

Obesity is the most potent risk factor for Type 2 diabetes, accounting for up to 85% of the overall risk of developing Type 2 diabetes, hence the current global spread of this metabolic condition. Your risk of diabetes is greater if there is already diabetes in the family, by race (six times more common in people of South Asian descent and up to three times more common among people of African and African-Caribbean origin), and occurrence also increases with age. Diagnosed conditions such as hypertension and polycystic ovary syndrome also increase the risk of diabetes, as does poor blood glucose regulation diagnosed as impaired fasting glycaemia or impaired glucose tolerance, which both indicate high blood glucose levels (hyperglycaemia). Other conditions such as raised triglycerides (fats in the blood) and some mental health problems can also elevate your risk, and the risk is also increased if you have had a stroke or heart attack.

There are several lifestyle factors under your control that can heighten your risk of diabetes:

- Excess body weight, particularly around the middle
- Eating too many sugary foods and refined carbohydrate foods
- Consuming too many calories from any type of food
- Drinking too much alcohol
- Smoking

The more risk factors that apply to you, the greater your risk of developing diabetes and other conditions with impaired blood glucose control.

'Optimum nutrition is the medicine of tomorrow'
Dr. Linus Pauling.

Type 1 diabetes

Type 1 diabetes (also known as insulin-dependent or juvenile diabetes) is less common than Type 2 diabetes mellitus. It is caused by an autoimmune disease resulting in permanent destruction of the beta cells in the pancreas, meaning that the body can no longer produce insulin and this has to be taken via injection or medication. Type 1 diabetes is usually diagnosed in childhood, although a series of studies have reported a consistent global rise in the incidence of Type 1 diabetes, thought to be due to environmental factors.

An autoimmune disease is one where the immune system attacks the body's own tissues, and is thought to be triggered by a virus or infection. However, once the immune system has dealt with the virus, it continues to destroy body tissues, as in rheumatoid arthritis. Although the symptoms of Type 1 diabetes can be affected by diet and exercise, it cannot be reversed or cured, and blood glucose regulation relies upon regular insulin injections.

Type 2 diabetes

This is also called non-insulin-dependent diabetes mellitus, and was previously known as adult-onset or late-onset diabetes, although with increasing levels of obesity it is increasingly diagnosed in young adults and children. In Type 2 diabetes, either the pancreas does not produce enough insulin to reduce blood glucose levels, or the insulin fails to have the required effect upon the cells, so blood glucose is not reduced. Therefore, characteristics of this disease include insulin deficiency and/or insulin resistance, with the result of hyperinsulinaemia (too much insulin in the blood stream), and hyperglycaemia (high blood glucose levels). Type 2 diabetes can often be controlled with diet and exercise, but if blood glucose levels fail to be stabilized, various medications and eventually insulin therapy are used.

Increased adiposity (especially around the middle) is associated with a state of chronic inflammation, which can eventually make cells dysfunctional, including an inability to respond to insulin (insulin resistance). In the current obesity crisis, fuelled by the UK's love of carbohydrate bakery goods such as biscuits, cakes, bread and pizza, this dysfunctional metabolism is extremely common. In addition to being a precursor to Type 2 diabetes, it also affects cholesterol metabolism, is associated with increased occurrence of arthritis and gout, fatty liver, cardiovascular disease and some cancers.

Insulin resistance

Many Type 2 diabetics, and those with pre-diabetes and metabolic syndrome suffer from a condition known as insulin resistance, where insulin is still released from the pancreas, but the cells do not respond to it. If insulin cannot 'open the gates' to enable glucose to enter body cells, glucose remains in the blood stream and creates hyperglycaemia (high blood sugar). Because the blood glucose levels remain high, the pancreas may continue to produce insulin, leading to hyperinsulinaemia (high blood insulin levels).

How insulin enables glucose to leave the blood stream and enter the cells

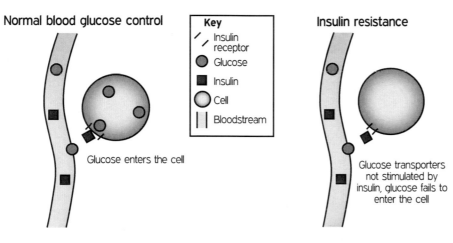

In normal insulin action, insulin causes a reaction at the cell membrance that allows glucose to enter the cell

In insulin resistance the glucose transporters in the cell do not allow glucose to enter the cell

Normal blood glucose control

Key

/ Insulin receptor

● Glucose

■ Insulin

○ Cell

| | Bloodstream

Glucose enters the cell

Insulin resistance

Glucose transporters not stimulated by insulin, glucose fails to enter the cell

Insulin resistance causes several health risks:

- It causes high blood glucose which results in blood proteins becoming glycated (denatured) by the excess glucose, rendering them useless

- Prolonged periods of hyperglycaemia also damage the lining of blood vessels, leading to many of the complications linked to diabetes

- Insulin supports the synthesis of lipoprotein lipase, an enzyme that breaks down triglycerides into fatty acids and glycerol, and facilitates storage of the fatty acids in adipocytes (fat cells). In the presence of insulin resistance, production of this enzyme is reduced, so fats cannot be moved into the cells, increasing fat deposition in other organs and elevating circulating levels of triglycerides and increasing the risk of cardiovascular disease

- Insulin resistance interferes with cholesterol metabolism, resulting in reduced levels of high density lipoprotein and therefore higher levels of cholesterol in the blood stream

- This increase in substances in the blood stream results in elevated blood pressure
- It also increases inflammation and the tendency to form blood clots.

Metabolic syndrome

Metabolic syndrome is the combination of diabetes, high blood pressure and obesity, also called insulin resistance syndrome because one of the features is high insulin levels and insulin resistance. It is very common and becoming more so, and contributory factors are being overweight, inactivity and a genetic predisposition.

Regulate your blood sugar through your diet

'25% of adults in the UK, and 35% in the United States have metabolic syndrome.'

The food and drink that we consume every day affects our blood glucose levels and can be either helpful or detrimental to blood glucose control. There are a number of ways you can adapt your diet to help regulate your blood sugar levels:

- Reduce your overall calorie intake to help maintain a healthy weight
- Reduce your intake of sugars and starchy carbohydrates
- Use the GI and GL of foods to stabilse blood glucose levels
- Reduce the amount of refined carbohydrates in your diet as this stimulates greater insulin release
- Include fish and vegetable proteins, but limit animal proteins
- Eat foods high in fibre that tend to contain a lower amount of starch and slow down glucose release into the blood stream
- Eat plenty of vegetables and some fruit for nutrients that can counteract oxidation and inflammation
- Limit alcohol intake
- Use spices such as cinnamon, which have proven anti-hyperglycaemic properties.

As all these dietary adjustments will affect blood glucose levels, if you are insulin dependent or using other medication that lowers blood glucose levels, you will need to work with your healthcare provider to adjust your medication prescription when embarking upon such dietary adjustments.

Control your weight, control your blood sugar levels

Obese people are over 80% more likely to become diabetic than someone with a healthy body mass index. Over 80% of people diagnosed with Type 2 diabetes are overweight. The more overweight and the more inactive you are, the greater your risk of Type 2 diabetes, particularly if the excess body fat is around the middle (abdominal obesity). Central obesity decreases our liver cells' sensitivity to insulin (the hormone that reduces blood glucose levels), and if the liver fails to take in glucose and store it, blood glucose levels remain elevated and the glucose is turned into fat (lipogenesis), increasing adipose levels even further.

Insulin promotes liver fat accumulation: during insulin resistance, even when insulin signaling for glucose metabolism is impaired, insulin signaling for fat metabolism is intact as the metabolic pathways are different, so excess glucose or amino acids can be turned into fat, less fat is used for energy, and fat deposition is increased. Excess fat deposition in the liver is present before the onset of classical Type 2 diabetes, and in established Type 2 diabetes, liver fat is always elevated. You can find out if you are at increased risk by checking your waist circumference or waist: hip ratio.

A number of studies and specific diet programmes have illustrated that Type 2 diabetes can be reversed with either low calorie or low carbohydrate intake. Restoration of normal glucose metabolism within days after bariatric surgery in the majority of people with Type 2 diabetes illustrates that a reversal of diabetes can be achieved with a profound decrease in food intake (Dixon *et al*, 2008; Pories *et al*, 1987).

Professor Roy Taylor and his team at Newcastle University have demonstrated that subjects following a very low calorie diet (800 calories daily for 8 weeks) exhibited normal glucose levels, and normal pancreatic function was restored, leading them to claim that 'diabetes can be reversed' (Taylor, 2012). The researchers' hypothesis is that chronic calorie excess leads to accumulation of liver fat and pancreatic fat, which causes insulin resistance in the liver and metabolic inhibition of pancreatic insulin secretion, causing hyperglycaemia. The study participants returned to normal eating following advice on healthy eating and improved portion control, and most were able to maintain their non-diabetic state.

The researchers also published the results of people following a very low calorie diet and reporting the same beneficial changes in weight, blood glucose, HbA1c, blood lipids and medication reduction. A clinical study to test the hypothesis, that very low calorie intake could reverse Type 2 diabetes, was funded by Diabetes.co.uk, with a mean weight loss of 15kg over eight weeks, and the same diabetes 'reversal' results (Lim *et*

'The 'apple' shape is less desirable than the 'pear' shape as far as health goes: adipose tissue around the abdomen is linked with increased risk of Type 2 diabetes, coronary heart disease and inflammatory endocrine disorders.'

al, 2011), and other researchers have found similar results using very low calorie diets. You can follow guidelines for a low calorie diet via Diabetes.co.uk. The NHS defines a low calorie diet as 1,000-1,500 calories per day for women / 1,500-2,000 calories per day for men, and a very low calorie diet is defined as a calorie intake of 1,000 calories or less per day. Very low calorie diets are viewed as extreme, and you should consult a suitably qualified healthcare practitioner to embark upon such a programme.

The extent of weight loss required to reverse Type 2 diabetes is much greater than usually advised. Moderate weight loss will improve glucose control but blood glucose levels and pancreatic function can remain abnormal. The Belfast diet study (1980) illustrated that a mean weight loss of 11kg lead to reasonably controlled, yet persistent diabetes. Data from the Swedish randomized study of gastric banding (Dixon *et al*, 2008) showed that a loss of 20% body weight was associated with long-term remission in 73% of a bariatric surgery group. Involuntary food shortage, such as during war, results in a sharp fall in Type 2 diabetes prevalence.

If you are a Type 1 diabetic balancing insulin medication with carbohydrate intake (carbohydrate units), it is still important to avoid over-eating and consumption of too much carbohydrate. Insulin is an anabolic hormone, so although it can reduce blood glucose levels (if there is no insulin resistance present), it simultaneously increases the formation of adipose tissue, and reduces lipolysis (break down of fat for energy). It is not healthy to consume too many carbohydrate foods and then medicate with insulin to deal with the resulting hyperglycaemia. Type 1 diabetics can also gain benefits in general health and weight loss from moderating carbohydrate and overall calorie intake, with a corresponding reduction in insulin. Good glycaemic control has been documented in Type 1 diabetic patients following a very low carbohyrdrate diet (Lennerz *et al*, 2018).

> 'Losing less than 1 gram of fat from the pancreas through diet can re-start the normal production of insulin, reversing Type 2 diabetes',
>
> Professor Roy Taylor

The effects of a low carbohydrate diet

Researchers Tay *et al* (2015) conducted a study comparing the effects of different amounts of carbohydrate in reduced calorie diets on weight, blood glucose and blood lipid parameters. Participants did three 1 hour exercise sessions weekly, and were monitored over one year. The proportions of macronutrients were:

Low carb diet: 14% of energy as carbohydrate (<50 g/day), 28% of energy as protein, and 58% of energy as fat (<10% saturated fat)

Higher carb diet: 53% of energy as carbohydrate, 17% of energy as protein, and 30% of energy as fat (<10% saturated fat).

The low carb group lost an average of 9.8 kg versus 10.1 kg in the higher carb group; HbA1c reduced by 1.0% in both groups, fasting glucose fell by 0.7 mmol/l in the low carb group and by 1.5 mmol/l in the higher carb group. The low carb group achieved greater mean reductions in diabetes medication. Both diets achieved substantial weight loss and reduced HbA1c and fasting glucose. The low carbohydrate diet, which was high in unsaturated fat and low in saturated fat, achieved greater improvements in the lipid profile (cholesterol, triglycerides), blood glucose stability, and reductions in diabetes medication requirements.

In a further study in 2018, Tay *et al* examined whether a low carbohydrate, high fat diet improved glycaemic control in overweight and obese patients with Type 2 diabetes compared with a high carbohydrate diet – both diets contained the same amount of energy and were low calorie diets.

- The low carb group lost an average of 6.8kg; the higher carb group lost 6.6kg
- The low carb group lost 4.3kg body fat, the high carb group lost an average of 4.6kg
- Fasting glucose in the low carb group fell by 0.3 mmol/l; the high carb group reduced fasting glucose levels by 0.4 mmol/l)
- The low carb group achieved greater reductions in diabetes medication use.

They concluded that both diets achieved comparable weight loss and HbA1c reductions. The lower carbohydrate group sustained greater reductions in diabetes medication requirements, and in improvements in blood glucose stability. However, these results suggest limited benefits from a lower carbohydrate intake.

It appears that a reduced energy intake is effective in reducing both weight (an independent risk factor for diabetes), and blood glucose parameters, although insulin levels were not measured in either of the aforementioned studies. With similar results in diets containing different amounts of carbohydrate, the overall effects on health might be considered. Jung and Choi (2017) reviewed studies done with Type 2 diabetic patients following various diets. They concluded that although higher carbohydrate diets are at least as effective as low carbohydrate diets regarding weight loss, reduced plasma glucose, HbA1c and low density lipoprotein cholesterol levels, high carbohydrate diets may raise serum triglyceride levels and reduce HDL (good) cholesterol (HDL-C), increasing the risk of cardiovascular disease. These effects did not always occur, and can be ameliorated by consuming low GI, low GL and high fibre foods, but if the effects upon weight loss and glucose metabolism are similar in low- or higher carbohydrate diets, yet there are cardiovascular benefits to eating fewer carbohydrates, it makes sense to reduce carbohydrate intake.

Moderating carbohydrate intake

As carbohydrates are formed from sugars such as glucose, the less carbohydrate you eat, the less glucose you will absorb into the bloodstream. This in itself will help to reduce blood glucose levels, and reduce the amount of insulin required to control blood glucose. However, carbohydrates are an important part of the diet, providing energy, fibre and essential nutrients, so it's important to keep some healthy carbohydrates in your diet.

There is more glucose in a starchy carbohydrate than in a non-starch carbohydrate (NSP), so reduce your intake of starchy carbohydrates but fill up on low GI fruits and vegetables containing less starch (and therefore less glucose). Many studies have shown a reduced risk of Type 2 diabetes with consumption of vegetables and some fruit. This is not only due to the reduced carbohydrate load, but also increased fibre and magnesium, and the protective anti-oxidant effects of vitamin C, vitamin E, carotenoids and flavonoids.

Follow these guidelines to get your carbohydrate intake right:

- Limit portion sizes of starchy carbohydrates such as rice, pasta, cereals and potatoes
- Eat moderate portions of low GI beans, pulses and lentils
- Fill up on non-starch carbohydrates such as salad and vegetables
- Choose lower GI fruits and vegetables to reduce glucose intake
- Avoid or limit foods with a high GI, particularly sugary foods and refined carbohydrates such as biscuits, cakes, muffins and pastries.

Making changes like these will increase nutrient intake whilst decreasing calories and carbohydrate intake. Here are some examples of how to adjust your meals to successfully reduce carbohydrate intake.

What to reduce	What to add in
Reduce your portion size of cereal	Add any low GI fruit – cherries, citrus fruits, apple, pear, cherries, prunes or strawberries...
Reduce your portion of rice	Add vegetables to the rice whilst it cooks, risotto-style. Pack it out with onions, garlic, frozen peas, peppers and sweet corn. Alternatively, cook the rice separately but add extra vegetables to the other part of your meal, packing out chili, curry or stroganoff with vegetables containing less starch and fewer calories.
Reduce your portion of pasta	Replace starchy pasta with water-rich aubergines, courgettes, tomatoes, red onions and garlic for a lower calorie and tastier Mediterranean style meal with added health benefits. If eating spaghetti or linguine, you can replace some or all of the pasta with spiralized or grated courgette, carrot, squash or sweet potato.
Have fewer potatoes	Swap potatoes for other vegetables. The bright colours of vegetables such as pumpkin, carrot, beetroot or broccoli denotes the high levels of phytonutrients in these foods, which all contain less starch and fewer calories than potatoes. You can also make mash with carrot, turnip, sweet potato or celeriac.

Using the GI or GL of foods to stabilize blood glucose levels

There are a number of ways that you can use the GI of foods to help stabilize blood glucose levels.

Avoiding and reducing the effect of high GI foods

You can avoid or limit foods with a high GI, eat smaller portions of high GI foods, and/ or combine these foods with low GI foods, proteins or fatty foods to slow down the absorption of glucose into your blood stream. Check out *Collins gem 'GI',* a handbag sized GI dictionary, arranged in food groups and listing foods in a traffic light style: red for high GI, amber for medium GI and green for low GI.

Swapping high GI for low GI foods

Simply swapping high GI foods for higher fibre, lower GI options can make a difference to blood sugar regulation. See how many of these you can do...

- Swap white bread to whole meal or GI bread

- Swap white rice to brown rice

- Swap white pasta for durum wheat pasta

- Replace some of your starchy carbohydrates with nutrient-rich lower carbohydrate non-starch polysaccharides (fruit and vegetables)

- Make cakes, muffins, pancakes and biscuits with less white flour and sugar – use more fruit, ground almonds or whole meal flour instead.

Swapping starchy carbohydrates for non-starch polysaccharides will also decrease your calorie intake and help you to control your weight, as well as increase the amount of anti-oxidants such as vitamin C and beta carotene, which help to counteract the damage done by the inflammation encountered in diabetes and heart disease.

We are more likely to eat a large portion of carbohydrate-rich foods than protein or fatty foods, as carbohydrates are usually very palatable and quicker to digest, particularly low fibre, refined carbohydrates such as white bread. Simply weighing the portion size of cereal, rice or pasta can help you to reduce the carbohydrate intake and produce less insulin. In reducing the portion size of carbohydrate foods, you are reducing the glycaemic load (GL) of your meal.

'Allow 30g of cereal for breakfast, and 60g of uncooked rice or pasta for a main meal.'

Manipulating the GI of your meals

Carbohydrate absorption and digestion is affected by lots of different factors…

- Eating high fibre foods slows down the absorption of glucose, resulting in lower blood glucose and insulin levels

- Combining lower GI or GL foods with high GI/GL foods will reduce the overall GI and GL of your meal

- Even if a food has a high GI, if you reduce the portion size you reduce the GL, so the amount of glucose you are consuming is lower

- Cooking foods for longer helps to break down the walls of the starch molecules – this makes the energy (glucose) more readily available and increases the GI, so al dente vegetables will be absorbed slower than vegetables cooked for a longer time.

Protein consumption and glycaemic control

Contrary to popular belief that eating proteins with carbohydrates may slow down the release of sugars into the bloodstream, research studies show that this doesn't happen, and that because the amino acids in protein also stimulate insulin release, insulin levels can be even higher if protein is added to a meal containing carbohydrates.

It seems that the beneficial effects of dietary protein on insulin secretion and glycemic control initially seen in high protein diets do not seem to persist long-term. Several studies addressing the association between protein intake and Type 2 diabetes have found an increased risk of diabetes with high protein and/or meat protein intake. Two large studies with >35,000 participants (Sluijs *et al*, 2010) observed a 30% increased risk of Type 2 diabetes with higher consumption of both total protein intake and animal protein intake, though there was no association with vegetable protein intake. The increased risk was present when protein was increased at the expense of, rather than in addition to, carbohydrate or fat, so there was not an overall calorie increase.

Research suggests that the type of protein could be of relevance. Type 2 diabetes risk is associated with higher meat consumption, particularly red and processed meat. Type 2 diabetes risk is reportedly lower in subjects with high dairy intake and/or high plant product consumption, especially legumes and nuts, and a recent study in the EPIC-InterAct case cohort reported no association between fish consumption and Type 2 diabetes (Patel *et al*, 2012).

In the largest study to date on protein intake and Type 2 diabetes, researchers agreed that high animal protein exchanged for carbohydrate intake was associated with a slightly higher risk of Type 2 diabetes, and that plant protein intake was not associated with increased risk (van Nielen *et al*, 2014). Type 2 diabetes incidence was 38% higher in women with the highest animal protein intake compared with women with the lowest intake, and the incidence increased 9% per 10g increment of animal protein intake. In obese women, the association was even stronger, with a risk increase of 19% for every additional 10g animal protein intake. In men, only a weak non-significant association was present.

How does dietary protein increase the risk of Type 2 diabetes?

Although carbohydrate intake is the main stimulant for insulin release, proteins also stimulate insulin release. Proteins are made up of amino acids, and different amino acids stimulate either insulin or glucagon secretion. Glucagon is a hormone secreted from the pancreas in response to low blood glucose levels; it generally has the opposing role to insulin, and stimulates the breakdown of stored carbohydrate (glycogen) back into glucose, and also stimulates the conversion of non-carbohydrate glucogenic amino acids, lactic acid and glycerol into glucose when glucose levels are very low. Hence, the action of glucagon is to raise blood glucose levels.

As some amino acids increase glucagon secretion, this is one way in which blood glucose levels may be elevated from consuming more protein. In the absence of diabetes, a rise in blood amino acid concentration stimulates the secretion of both glucagon and insulin, so blood glucose remains stable. The insulin is secreted to enable amino acid uptake and stimulate protein synthesis in muscle cells, and the glucagon is secreted to stimulate the uptake of amino acids into the cells of the liver for gluconeogenesis. The release of insulin ensures that the amino acids are used for protein synthesis and the glucagon ensures that blood sugar doesn't drop to dangerously low levels, even if the meal was low in carbohydrate. However, in people with diabetes, the release of glucagon with impaired insulin response can cause blood sugar to rise precipitously several hours after a meal high in protein.

Different amino acids stimulate secretion of insulin and glucagon

Arginine stimulates the highest secretion of both insulin and glucagon. The amino acids known to stimulate glucagon secretion are glutamine and ornithine. Amino acids more prone to increase insulin secretion are leucine, isoleucine, alanine, and arginine. Foods containing high amounts of these amino acids will incite higher insulin levels, possibly leading to hyperinsulinemia, a risk factor for insulin resistance. Lin *et al* (2000) compared the insulin and glucagon secretion in groups consuming high and moderate protein intake over six months. They found that insulin secretion was increased in the high protein group (average 516 pmol/l versus 305 pmol/l). Endogeneous glucose output (glucose formation from the liver) was increased by 12% in the high protein group, probably due to increased glucagon secretion, as gluconeogenesis was also increased by 40%. Fasting plasma glucagon was 34% increased in the high protein group. They concluded that high protein intake is accompanied by increased stimulation of glucagon and insulin.

Different types of protein affect insulin response

Among healthy people, consuming protein with carbohydrate typically increases the insulin response and reduces blood sugar. However, one study reports that in those with Type 2 diabetes, combining protein with carbohydrate increased after-meal insulin levels, but reduced insulin action so the ability of insulin to move glucose from the bloodstream to the body tissues was compromised, leading to elevated blood sugar (Ang *et al*, 2012). They also found that the differing absorption times of different types of proteins affected insulin response and insulin action. A fast absorbing protein such as whey or soya protein reduced insulin action to a greater extent than a slow-absorbing protein such as casein, so proteins that are absorbed more quickly are not recommended for those with Type 2 diabetes. This may partially explain the link between higher protein intake and increased risk of Type 2 diabetes.

Several mechanisms may explain the relationship between protein intake and diabetes.

1 Some amino acids can reduce insulin action causing high blood glucose levels, continued release of insulin and potentially create insulin resistance.

2 Amino acids also stimulate glucagon secretion, which increases blood glucose levels through breaking down glycogen (to release additional glucose into the blood stream), and gluconeogenesis (making new glucose). Although insulin is meant to prevent high glucose levels, in Type 2 diabetes or pre-diabetes a person may have impaired insulin secretion.

3 A further option is that iron metabolism may be involved. Iron overload is associated with increased diabetes risk, and animal proteins are often rich in iron. However, this association with insulin sensitivity requires further research

4 Other research suggests that nitrites and advanced glycation end-products (formed from browning foods during grilling, frying, roasting, baking) may also play a role in the development of Type 2 diabetes. These products are most often found in conjunction with processed meat products.

How to moderate protein intake to help regulate blood glucose levels

Different proteins are digested and absorbed at different rates, and the amino acids (which make up proteins) that stimulate glucagon are different from those that stimulate insulin secretion. As proteins also stimulate insulin release, the insulin response after a meal containing carbohydrate and protein can be as high as carbohydrate intake alone – the key thing is to reduce overall food intake to limit insulin secretion and storage of excess nutrients. Although a higher protein intake has positive effects on satiety and increasing energy expenditure through thermogenesis and increased lean tissue metabolism, it can have detrimental effects on glucose homeostasis by promoting insulin resistance and increasing gluconeogenesis. Adjusting the type of protein foods consumed rather than the quantity of proteins is more beneficial to insulin metabolism, with fish and vegetable proteins possibly having the most desirable effects on insulin sensitivity. Additionally, consuming a little more protein and less carbohydrate in a hypo-calorific diet is beneficial, but if energy consumption is maintaining current weight or increasing body weight, a higher protein intake is associated with increased Type 2 diabetes risk.

Using protein foods to your advantage

In a review of the effects of overeating different amounts of carbohydrates, fats and protein, Leaf and Antonio (2017) found that weight gain (fat gain) was less in those over-consuming protein when compared to overconsumption of carbohydrate and fat, between which there was little difference. The main effect of protein upon energy balance is related to increased satiety – protein takes longer to digest than other types of food, so it makes us feel fuller for longer. High-protein diets seem to be positively associated with weight loss, with favourable body composition and metabolism changes. This is thought to be due to the following:

- Increased satiety, leading to lower calorie consumption
- A higher thermogenic effect, so the net amount of energy from each gram of protein is less than from other macronutrients
- Improvements in body composition – a greater amount of lean muscle results in a higher metabolic rate and therefore increased energy expenditure.

So here are some ways to utilize protein in your diet without increasing your risk of Type 2 diabetes:

- Eat protein instead of carbohydrate rather than adding protein to meals, so that you are not increasing the total calorie density of the meal, and not increasing overall insulin release
- Choose fish or vegetable proteins (nuts, beans, lentils, chickpeas) over meat, especially red and processed meats.

Protein helps to increase satiety and reduce calorie intake by making you feel full, reducing the likelihood of eating sugary snacks between meals. The resultant reduction in calorie intake and lower body fat levels will reduce the risk of inflammation and damage to insulin receptive cells, the cause of insulin resistance and Type 2 diabetes.

'Grab a handful of protein-rich, low GI nuts as a snack between meals to boost energy levels. Be careful if you're watching your calorie intake though, as nuts are a concentrated source of energy.'

The actions of normal, healthy insulin secretion is positive, as it reduces blood glucose levels. However, if too many calories are consumed, insulin promotes fat storage and weight gain. The other key issue is that when adipose levels are high, the resulting inflammation affects insulin responsive cells – they become insulin resistant and glucose cannot be absorbed into the cells, causing hyperglycaemia and hyperinsulinaemia.

The effects of fats upon glucose metabolism

High intake of saturated and trans fats may contribute to the development of diabetes via obesity, although several studies suggest that higher intake of unsaturated fats found in fish, nuts, seeds, avocado, olives and vegetable oils could reduce the risk of Type 2 diabetes. Although fat slows down the emptying of the stomach and the absorption of sugar into the bloodstream, it doesn't seem to reduce insulin secretion. Montonen at al (2015) reviewed the diet and incidence of diabetes in over 4000 men and women, and found that eating poultry, vegetable oils and margarine were linked to a lower risk. Trans fats and some saturated fats may alter the structure of cell membranes to inhibit insulin binding and glucose absorption. Different types of fats appear to have varying effects upon insulin sensitivity and glucose absorption. The best types of fats appear to be those found in vegetable sources such as vegetable oils, nuts, seeds, avocado, olives and coconut.

Moderate alcohol consumption

Alcohol affects blood glucose levels and can increase your risk of Type 2 diabetes in a number of ways. Some types of alcoholic beverage such as wine and beer contain sugar, elevating blood sugar levels, but excess alcohol can actually cause hypoglycaemia (low blood glucose), stimulating the appetite, causing overeating and poor food choices. Alcohol reduces the blood glucose level as it affects the liver's ability to release stored glucose into the bloodstream. Alcohol intake may also increase blood pressure and triglyceride levels and it contains 7 calories per gram, so also contributes to weight gain – all risk factors for Type 2 diabetes.

Cullmann *et al* (2012) reported that total alcohol consumption and binge drinking increased the risk of pre-diabetes and Type 2 diabetes in men, but low consumption decreased diabetes risk in women. High consumption of spirits increased the risk in both men and women. In a large-scale meta-analysis, Knott *et al* (2012) concluded that reductions in Type 2 diabetes risk due to moderate alcohol intake might be confined to women and non-Asian populations. However, a review by Huang *et al* in 2017 reported a U-shaped relationship between wine, beer or spirits and Type 2 diabetes. Wine consumption was associated with a significant risk reduction, and the peak risk reduction was 20-30 g/day for wine and beer, and at 7-15 g/day for spirits, with a decrease of 20% (wine), 9% (beer) and 5% (spirits). This risk reduction equates to approximately 2 units of wine or beer, and one unit of spirits.

Most guidelines for those with diabetes, or to reduce your risk of diabetes, involve moderating alcohol intake.

- Limit alcohol consumption to no more than two units daily, stay within the recommended guidelines of 14 units weekly, and have several alcohol free days each week

- It seems that the best option if you are going to drink alcohol is wine, followed by beer and then spirits. Red wine may offer some additional anti-oxidant/anti-inflammatory benefits through its polyphenol content

- If you are going to drink alcohol, don't' drink it on its own as it will affect blood glucose levels more severely. Drink it shortly before, during or soon after a meal

- Do not substitute alcoholic drinks for your usual meal or snacks as this may lead to hypoglycaemia, particularly if you already have difficulties controlling blood sugar levels

- Serious hypoglycaemia can occur with larger quantities of alcohol, particularly if you are treated with insulin and if too little carbohydrate is eaten, so always eat some starchy carbohydrates with alcohol

- Low carbohydrate beers and cider have a higher alcohol content which contains more calories and is more likely to cause hypoglycaemia

- Low alcohol wines are often higher in sugar than ordinary wine, so this is not necessarily a good option

- Drinks with high sugar content such as sweet wines, 'Alco pops' and liqueurs should be limited due to the high sugar and calorie count.

Coffee and Type 2 diabetes

The most recent epidemiological and research data suggests that long-term consumption of coffee is associated with a lower risk of developing Type 2 diabetes in healthy individuals (Rebelo and Casal, 2017). Other caffeinated beverages such as tea or energy drinks do not appear to provide the same therapeutic effect on diabetes risk, so additional factors must contribute to coffee's therapeutic nature. There are many constituents within the coffee beverage, and it is thought that antioxidant activity and anti-inflammatory effects may be partially responsible for this therapeutic effect.

However, when we consume caffeinated products, our adrenal glands produce adrenaline. Adrenaline is our 'fight or flight' hormone, and stimulates the conversion of stored carbohydrate back into glucose, elevating blood sugar levels. This is what creates the energy surge that you experience when you have a cup of tea or coffee, or a glass of caffeinated cola. We often use caffeine to improve our energy levels, but it can, if used too frequently, also result in energy slumps in between 'fixes', so limit your coffee intake to two to three cups daily. It is interesting to note that Bhupathiraju *et al* (2013) reported that coffee intake reduced the risk of Type 2 diabetes, but caffeine-free coffee with artificial sweeteners was associated with an increased risk.

Other healthy alternatives

Various herbs and spices can help you to control blood glucose levels. By replacing your usual brew with one of these drinks, you are not only reducing the blood sugar highs from caffeine stimulation, but are actually helping to improve your blood glucose control. Try some of these alternatives:

- Green tea contains catechins which have strong anti-oxidant properties and have been shown to improve pancreatic function
- Place a cinnamon stick into some hot water or milk to enjoy the anti-hyperglycaemic properties of cinnamon
- Sage tea has been shown to reduce blood glucose and have metformin-like effects.

Sweeteners

Recent research has discovered that sweeteners containing no sugar can still incite an insulin response. This is because part of the stimulus for insulin release is via the nervous system involved with digestion – when we eat something sweet, our brain registers this and stimulates insulin release, regardless of the amount of glucose in the blood stream, although blood glucose levels are a strong stimulus for insulin secretion. Recent studies have shown an association between consumption of sweeteners and increased risk of Type 2 diabetes (Imamura *et al*, 2015).

Spices and herbs with anti-hyperglycaemic properties

There are a number of spices and herbs that are believed to help control blood glucose levels, such as cinnamon, fenugreek and turmeric. Each spice or herb reduces blood glucose levels in different ways – it is thought that the phenol and polyphenol compounds

'The anti-oxidant activity of green tea catechins is 25 to 100 times more powerful than vitamins C and E.'

in spices might affect either absorption of glucose in the intestine, insulin secretion, glucose production in the liver, or cellular glucose uptake. Most importantly, they have the potential to help you control your blood sugar levels, and are tasty, nutritious and easy to add to your diet, providing a healthy alternative to added sugar or sweeteners.

Add cinnamon to...

- Porridge and other cereals
- Puddings such as rice pudding or bread and butter pudding
- Baked or stewed fruit
- Hot drinks such as herbal teas or hot chocolate – add a cinnamon stick or sprinkle in some of the spice.

Add turmeric to...

- Curries, chilies, stews and casseroles
- Stir fry, baked or roasted meats, fish or vegetables
- Sauces or salad dressings
- Yoghurt to make your own dip.

Add fenugreek seeds to...

- Curries or chilies
- Stir fries
- Roasted or baked vegetables, meats or fish, sprinkling them on top
- Salads.

'Whilst definitive conclusions cannot be drawn regarding the therapeutic use of cinnamon as an anti-diabetic therapy, there is little doubt regarding its anti-hyperglycaemic effects.'

Supplements

Chromium

Jamilian *et al* (2018) conducted a randomized double-blind, placebo-controlled trial with 40 women taking either 200 mcg/day of chromium or placebo for 8 weeks. The chromium supplement led to significant reductions in fasting plasma glucose, insulin levels, insulin resistance, serum triglycerides and total cholesterol when compared with the placebo, and was also associated with a significant increase in plasma antioxidant capacity.

Alpha lipoic acid (ALA)

Alpha lipoic acid is a powerful natural antioxidant. Trials indicate that supplementing 600 to 1,200 mg of ALA daily can improve insulin sensitivity and the symptoms of diabetic neuropathy. Best results have been seen from intravenous administration of ALA, but McIlduff and Rutkove (2011) report beneficial effects with an oral dose of 600 mg daily administered for up to 5 weeks.

Fibre supplements

Fibre supplements such as psyllium and fenugreek seeds have improved glucose tolerance in some studies. Fibre slows down glucose absorption, and fenugreek may also stimulate insulin production. 15g of powdered fenugreek seeds added to meals can reduce blood glucose levels, and taking 1 – 2.5g daily has shown beneficial results (Neelakantan et al, 2014). Gaddam et al (2015) found that 10g of fenugreek powder daily reduced the risk of Type 2 diabetes in pre-diabetic subjects. Those in the control group had a 4.2 times higher risk of developing diabetes compared to those consuming fenugreek. Forty Type 2 diabetes patients given psyllium fibre (10.5 g daily) significantly reduced BMI, fasting blood glucose, HbA1c and insulin levels, giving conclusive evidence that supplementation with this fibre can improve glucose metabolism in Type 2 diabetic patients.

Magnesium

People with Type 2 diabetes tend to have low magnesium levels, and magnesium supplementation has improved insulin production in some trials. In a systematic review associating dietary magnesium intake with risk of developing Type 2 diabetes, those with the highest magnesium consumption had a 17% lower risk. A statistically significant linear dose-response relationship was found between magnesium intake and diabetes risk, with risk reduced by 8%–13% per 100mg/day increment in dietary magnesium intake. This suggests a role for magnesium in prevention of Type 2 diabetes. Ideally, this should be provided by the diet with sufficient vegetables, nuts and pulses, but supplementation can also be considered.

Vitamin D

Evidence strongly suggests that vitamin D modifies the risk of Type 2 diabetes through effects upon the pancreas, insulin sensitivity and systemic inflammation. Most studies show an inverse association between vitamin D status and prevalence of Type 2 diabetes, although this is mostly based upon vitamin D levels in those with diabetes rather than studying the effects of vitamin D supplementation. Those with higher intakes and/or serum levels of vitamin D had up to a 40% lower risk of developing Type 2 diabetes. The potential effect of vitamin D appears to be more prominent among those at risk for diabetes (Mitri and Pittas, 2014).

Summing Up

To reduce the risk of diabetes and manage blood glucose metabolism:

- Reduce overall calorie consumption and maintain a healthy weight
- Limit your overall intake of carbohydrates
- Choose high fibre, low GI carbohydrates such as vegetables, oats and beans
- Include a little protein in small, regular meals throughout the day to improve satiety, but reduce other food groups to accommodate the added protein
- Choose fish and vegetable proteins over meat, especially red/processed meat
- Avoid trans fats and limit saturated fats in meats
- Limit alcohol consumption as this affects blood sugar control
- Drink coffee, green tea or make a cinnamon or turmeric infused milk
- Add herbs and spices such as cinnamon to your food to improve glucose metabolism and blood sugar control.

Stick to...	Stay away from...
Low GI foods	High GI foods
High fibre foods	Refined carbohydrates
Low starch vegetables	Excess carbohydrate, protein, fat
Coffee or green tea	Sweetened beverages
Protein at each meal	Fruit juices
Cinnamon and other anti-hyperglycaemic herbs and spices	Sugar and sweeteners

Food for thought

Although we automatically reach for food and drink to cheer us up, improve focus, or even help us get to sleep, not many people make the connection between mental function and their diet, and yet the two are closely linked. Why do you drink milk to help you sleep and coffee to perk you up? Why does chocolate cheer you up, and does fish really 'make you brainy'?!

One in six people have a mental health condition (NHS Digital, 2016), and an increasing amount of research is being done illustrating vital links between fatty acid deficiency and impaired cognitive (mental) function, with conditions such as dementia, attention deficit hyperactivity disorder, depression, anxiety, dyslexia and other mental health conditions often responding well to fatty acid supplementation and an improved diet.

We all have ups and downs, but whether your 'mood swings' or 'fuzzy brain' moments are passing or long term, there may be several dietary adjustments that can help.

Feeding your brain what it needs!

Whilst specific foods and nutrients have been linked with certain mental conditions, there is no doubt that what we consume affects how we feel and function. There are some fundamental dietary 'must do's' that affect mental health and performance. These are:

- Ensuring adequate hydration
- Balancing blood glucose levels
- Consuming a rainbow diet to provide all the phytonutrients and anti-oxidants we need for continued good health
- Consuming high quality protein and fatty foods such as fish, eggs and nuts.

Water

There is a well-established link between hydration and improved cognitive performance among adults and children. Adequate hydration is crucial for good health, and critical to mental and physical performance. The human body is over two-thirds water weight, and just 2% dehydration begins to affect our mental performance. Surveys have reported that less than 1% of people meet fluid intake recommendations, and 20% of GP visits are with symptoms such as tiredness, headaches and lack of energy, which can all be caused by dehydration.

The NHS Eat Well Guide states that we should drink six to eight glasses of fluid daily, but a more accurate guideline is based upon an individual's body weight. The Oxford Handbook of Nutrition and Dietetics (2012) recommends that we consume 35ml of fluid per kg body weight, but all of these recommendations are not taking account of the fluid in high water content fruit and vegetables, milk or soup. However, if your diet is not meeting the recommended 5 (to 10) portions of fruit and vegetables per day, what you eat is less likely to be contributing much to your fluid requirements.

Tips for meeting your fluid needs

- Start the day with a drink of hot water rather than a caffeinated drink, which stimulates urine production and therefore aids fluid loss. Add a squeeze of fresh lemon/lime, a chunk of cucumber or a drop of red grape juice if you need a little flavour

- Fill a 1.5 or 2 litre bottle and take keep it with you at work/home – drinking from this through the day gives you a measure of how much you've drunk, and having the bottle in front of you will remind you to drink regularly

- Keep smaller water bottles in the car or in your bag, so you are never caught out without water to hand

- Always drink more if you are exercising

- Sip fluids throughout the day – hydration is achieved more successfully in this way, rather than drinking a large amount quickly

- Fill a large jug of water at home and flavour it with chunks of cucumber, orange, lime or lemon to make you more likely to drink it

- Drink herbal or fruit teas through the day as these will hydrate you rather than act as diuretics like tea, coffee, hot chocolate and many energy drinks

- Alcohol is also a diuretic as it switches off the release of anti-diuretic hormone from the posterior pituitary gland, so you need to drink more water whenever you consume alcohol

- Consume foods with high water content such as fresh fruit (not dried) and vegetables.

Adequate hydration is achieved when the volume of urine produced matches fluid intake, or when the colour of urine is a pale straw colour – an easy way to monitor hydration levels!

Sugar and blood glucose regulation

A diet full of processed foods is lacking in the nutrients that we need to feed our brain, resulting in symptoms such as irritability, aggression, inability to concentrate and depression. Healthy blood glucose regulation is crucial for mental function and wellbeing. Low blood glucose can cause irritability, restlessness and poor concentration. Research with school children has shown improvements in attention, problem solving and memory when comparing the effect of breakfast versus no breakfast, although sugar rich cereals can create problems – in addition to being devoid of minerals and vitamins, added sugar creates fluctuations in blood glucose levels, contributing to hyperactivity, mood swings and poor concentration.

Meals with a lower glycaemic index (GI) help to balance blood glucose levels, avoiding low blood glucose (hypoglycaemia) and high blood glucose (hyperglycaemia). Carbohydrates with a lower GI include oats, most vegetables and pulses; high GI foods tend to contain more sugar or are more processed, such as white bread products and many breakfast cereals. Swapping refined carbohydrates for a protein-rich meal can be beneficial: although protein also induces insulin secretion, it tends to have balancing effect upon blood glucose levels, and will also provide many important micronutrients such as zinc and iron.

One 14-year study examining links between childhood diet and teenage anti-social behaviour illustrated a 51% rise in aggression at age 17 in those who ate a poor diet with low levels of zinc, iron, B vitamins and protein. These deficiencies were linked to poor brain development, which led to a low IQ, resulting in anti-social behaviour. In another study, IQ was found to be 25 points lower in children who ate a diet rich in refined carbohydrates (Food and Behaviour Research, 2018).

So for basic healthy mental function throughout the day, ensure you are adequately hydrated and blood glucose is balanced with nutrient-rich foods. Here is a sample menu to get you started.

A menu to maximize mental performance!

Breakfast options

Milky porridge with added mixed seeds, chopped walnuts and fruit
Omega 3 fortified boiled egg with toasted whole meal bread
Scrambled/poached egg on whole meal toast with baked beans and mushrooms

Lunch options

Tuna or salmon salad sandwich with whole meal bread
Corn tortilla wrap with turkey, spinach, bean sprouts and avocado
Sardines on whole meal toast with beetroot

Dinner options

Turkey or salmon risotto
Vegetable chilli with brown rice
Home made salmon or cod fish fingers with peas and sweet potato mash

Snacks

Pieces of fresh fruit – eat a variety of different fruits for a wide range of nutrients
Nut/seed mix
Nut or seed bar

Depression and Seasonal affective disorder

A depressed mood ranges from feeling low, through temporary conditions such as pre-menstrual syndrome or seasonal affective disorder, to long-term depression, and with such a wide range of causes, symptoms and conditions it is impossible to address them all individually here. Our mood is affected by the foods that we eat, so adjusting the diet is a good place to start. However, depression is a multifactorial disorder with different causes, so whilst some individuals with depression respond well to fatty acid or zinc supplementation, others may not. Whilst discovering blood serum levels of various vitamins, minerals and fatty acids is possible to establish causality, many of the dietary adjustments suggested herein would convey a general improvement in overall health for many individuals anyway, based upon typical levels of micronutrients and essential fatty acids.

'It has been suggested that approximately 70% of the population in Europe are deficient in vitamin D.'

Seasonal affective disorder

It's funny how a spell in the sunshine makes us feel happier and the winter months can lower mood; in those of us more susceptible to the change in seasons, this is diagnosed as seasonal affective disorder. We actually create most of the vitamin D in our bodies from being in sunlight, and several large scale studies have reported that vitamin D supplementation has an anti-depressant effect, with some researchers stating that depression increases when vitamin D levels dip below normal. Researchers have concluded that vitamin D deficiency may be associated with an increased risk or severity of depression. Although vitamin D is found in eggs, dairy foods, oily fish, fortified margarines and cereals, most of the vitamin D in the human body is formed from exposure to sunlight, so a little sunshine really can boost your mood.

Depression

Multiple research studies have shown that the risk of developing depression is directly linked to diet, lifestyle and exercise (Lopresti *et al*, 2013). Risk of depression is most closely linked to a poor diet, followed by physiological factors and then lifestyle patterns such as sleep and exercise. Research has shown that a diet comprised of fibre-rich foods such as leafy green salads, vegetables and whole grains has been consistently associated with a reduced risk for depression, and a diet high in processed foods and high fat dairy is associated with increased risk of depression.

Serotonin

Levels of 'feel good' hormones called endorphins can be lower in some individuals, causing moodiness, increased agitation and in some cases, depression. Women who experience changes in mood prior to or during menstruation (pre-menstrual syndrome (PMS)) have been found to have lower levels of serotonin in their brain, which can also increase sensitivity to pain. A common treatment for low mood or depression is a type of tranquilizer known as selective serotonin reuptake inhibitors (SSRIs), which are thought to inhibit the re-uptake of serotonin and enhance circulating serotonin levels. Selective serotonin re-uptake inhibitors account for 16 million NHS prescriptions a year.

However, in 2004, a review of published studies on SSRIs including previously hidden unpublished data was conducted to analyse research and compile British regulatory clinical guidelines. In adults with mild to moderate depression it was concluded that SSRIs are no better than placebo. In 2005, the British Medical Journal published another study that concluded that SSRIs are no more effective than a placebo and do not reduce depression, and it has been stated that only one in ten patients responds specifically to an SSRI rather than a placebo. In the largest study of its kind studying published and unpublished data on SSRIs, it was concluded that antidepressant drugs do not work (Kirsch *et al*, 2008). More than £291 million was spent on antidepressants in 2006, including nearly £120 million on SSRIs.

However, a countering study by Ciprani *et al* (2018) reviewed the published and unpublished data of over 500 trials, reporting the results after eight weeks of anti-depressant drugs versus placebo or comparing two different medicines. Prozac – now known by its generic name, fluoxetine – was one of the least effective but best tolerated, and amitriptyline seemed to be the most effective but had lower tolerance. They concluded that all the drugs were more effective than placebo for the short-term treatment of acute depression in adults. However, the result was actually no different to the earlier study stating that SSRIs are ineffective, there was simply a different slant on translating the evidence. Using standardized research measures of effect size, Kirsch *et al* stated an effect of 0.32 on a scale where 0.2 is considered small and 0.5 medium effect, Cipriani *et al* stated an even smaller effect of 0.30.

Serotonin-boosting foods

Serotonin, the 'feel good hormone', is a neurotransmitter, enabling chemical messages to travel around our brain. Serotonin is formed from an essential amino acid (found in protein foods) called tryptophan. The insulin released when we eat indirectly increases the amount of tryptophan taken up by the brain cells, enabling more serotonin formation, boosting our mood and helping us to relax, hence the 'happy, relaxed' feeling experienced after a big plate of pasta or bread, so eating carbohydrate foods with tryptophan-rich foods may boost your mood even more. Serotonin also initiates sleep.

Tryptophan-rich foods

- Turkey
- Chicken
- Avocados
- Bananas
- Broccoli
- Spinach.

Changing your food to affect your mood

Fatty acids

'There are significant correlations between worldwide fish consumption and rates of depression.'

Clinically depressed people often have lower levels of omega 3 fatty acids in their blood, and several studies have shown that supplementing a diet with omega 3 fatty acids can improve depression (Grosso *et al*, 2014). Eating more omega 3 fatty acids leads to a higher volume of grey matter in the areas of the brain associated with emotional arousal and regulation, and these fats also enhance mood. Higher consumption of seafood in some countries has been linked with protection against depression, bipolar disorder and seasonal affective disorder.

Other essential nutrients

Zinc

Several studies have linked psychological symptoms to low zinc levels; in one study of 174 older adults, 71% of subjects with zinc deficiency displayed a higher value on a depression test against 29% of subjects with a normal zinc value. Common symptoms of zinc deficiency can include the following…

- White specks on nails
- Stretch marks in the skin
- Poor blood sugar control
- Mood swings and depression.

The B vitamins

Symptoms affecting the brain and mental function have been linked with a number of the B vitamins, and several studies show improvements in mood following supplementation of all, or various B vitamins (White *et al*, 2015; Almeida *et al*, 2014; Skarupski *et al*, 2010). Relatively low levels of each of the B vitamins are required to maintain good health and these are found in a wide range of foods, usually occurring together. Make sure you base each meal around these foods and it is unlikely you will have a deficiency of B vitamins:

- Vegetables
- Whole grains
- Fruit
- Beans and pulses
- Eggs
- Meat
- Fish
- Dairy produce.

Vitamin B1 (thiamine) mimics and maximizes the action of an important neurotransmitter involved in memory function called acetylcholine. In several double-blind, placebo controlled studies, thiamine supplementation improved mood and feelings of wellbeing, with subjects also reporting increased clear-headedness and faster reaction times.

For vitamin B1...

- Add a seed mix to fortified cereals
- For a quick snack, eat beans on whole meal toast
- Enjoy mixed beans in chilies, curries and casseroles.

For more vitamin B12 ...

- Breakfast on eggs on toast
- Add tofu to stir fries
- Eat yoghurt for a healthy snack.

A number of studies have reported an association between deficiencies of vitamin B12 or folate and psychiatric conditions such as dementia and depression.

Folic acid (B9)

A high percentage of depressed patients have been found to have poor folic acid levels. Folic acid is involved in producing neurotransmitters, the chemical messengers in the brain, and without ample levels of neurotransmitters, our mental function quickly becomes impaired.

For more folic acid in your diet...

- Eat raspberries with fortified breakfast cereals
- Always add spinach, rocket or watercress to salad sandwiches
- Enjoy salads with salmon or cottage cheese.

Please note!

Many nutrients are involved in healthy mental function.

Therefore, rather than supplement with any one nutrient, it is recommended that unless you are following a treatment plan prescribed by a qualified practitioner, a multi-vitamin, multi-mineral supplement is the best way to increase nutrient intake alongside a healthy diet.

Attention deficit disorder, hyperactivity, dyslexia, autism...

Although these are all separate conditions, their occurrence often overlaps in families and in individuals, the conditions share many of the symptoms, and they often respond well to the same dietary adjustments. In particular, scientific evidence suggests that fatty acid deficiencies or imbalances may contribute to a wide range of behavioral and learning disorders.

ADHD

ADHD is estimated to affect up to 5% of school-aged children and up to 4% of adults in the UK. Standard pharmaceutical interventions for ADHD are often unsuccessful, and adverse effects are experienced in a third of pharmaceutical users, regardless of success of treatment. Clinical evidence suggests that deficiencies of polyunsaturated fatty acids could be related to ADHD – children and adolescents with the condition are consistently shown to have lower omega-3 blood levels and a higher omega-6/omega-3 ratio, and meta-analyses illustrate positive results following fatty acid supplementation in the management of ADHD symptoms.

Essential fatty acids

Essential fatty acids and long chain fatty acids are often lacking in our diet, and a high intake of saturated, trans and hydrogenated fats and even omega 6 fatty acids worsen our fatty acid balance even more. Research shows positive results in hyperactivity, anti-social behaviour and cognitive function following fatty acid supplementation, especially where a combination of long-chain omega 3 fatty acids and gamma-linolenic acid are taken together. Data from randomized controlled trials studying over 500 children and teens with ADHD has shown that omega-3 supplementation can significantly boost attention, cognition, and other ADHD-related challenges in children with attention deficit disorder. Symptoms of inattention and hyperactivity were significantly decreased when children were given an omega-3 supplement, compared to children who were given a placebo, and cognitive performance was also improved. One review states that the most promising results are found in trials where treatments combined omega 3 and omega 6 fatty acids (Königs and Kiliaan, 2016).

Whilst including fish in the diet will boost omega-3 intake, the therapeutic levels that can only be derived from supplementation may be needed for measurable changes in behavior or cognition, and a qualified health professional should be consulted.

Vitamin D

Patrick and Ames (2015) propose that because brain serotonin (our 'happy hormone') is synthesized from an amino acid called tryptophan, and this synthesis is activated by vitamin D, inadequate levels of vitamin D affect various aspects of mental function. The long chain fatty acids EPA and DHA are also required in this pathway, explaining why these nutrients may also improve cognition, mood and behaviour. Vitamin D therefore has a role in prevention, and possibly treatment of, ADHD, bipolar disorder, schizophrenia, and impulsive behavior.

Whole foods versus junk foods

A diet full of processed foods is lacking in the nutrients that we need to feed our brain, resulting in symptoms such as irritability, aggression, inability to concentrate and depression. In addition to being devoid of minerals and vitamins, added sugar also creates fluctuations in blood glucose levels, contributing to hyperactivity, mood swings and poor concentration.

In 2007 *The Food Magazine* reported that several colourings and preservatives regularly used in food and drinks would have to carry health warnings if they were added to medicines. Warnings include allergic and hyperactivity reactions for the following additives, which are commonly used in products such as cakes, sweets and soft drinks.

- Tartrazine
- Sunset yellow
- Ponceau red (all artificial colourings)
- Sodium benzoate
- Sodium dioxide
- Sodium metabisulphite (all preservatives).

Many additives are outlawed in other countries including the USA and Japan, but are still added to cheap, processed foods available in the UK despite numerous studies reporting that the behavior of hyperactive children improves when artificial food colourings are eliminated from their diet. The average improvement from eliminating these additives from the diet is around one third to one half of the improvement typically associated with medication for attention deficit hyperactivity disorder.

Not all additives are bad – some E numbers are natural compounds, such as anti-oxidant vitamin C (ascorbic acid), or curcumin derived from the yellow spice turmeric providing colouring to foods. Check out a full list of E numbers at **www.ukfoodguide.net/enumeric**.

For improved focus and attention...

- Avoid foods with artificial additives and a long list of E numbers as much as possible
- Stabilize blood sugar levels to avoid hypoglycaemia and lack of concentration (from low blood sugar) and hyperactivity (from high blood sugar) by introducing slow release carbohydrates such as porridge and beans into the diet
- Include protein foods such as eggs, fish or meat in each meal to help balance glucose regulation in the blood stream
- Eat fish or vegetable sources of alpha-linolenic acid (linseeds, walnuts) to provide a good source of long chain polyunsaturated fatty acids for the brain.

'Research with school children has shown improvements in attention, problem solving and memory when comparing the effect of breakfast versus no breakfast.'

Dementia and Alzheimer's disease

There are several different types of dementia, but the most common cause is Alzheimer's disease. Epidemiological evidence shows that our increased incidence of 'old-age' dementia and Alzheimer's has less to do with our increased life-expectancy and more to do with our diet causing increased adiposity and insulin resistance, which leads to disrupted neuronal insulin activity. This finding matches earlier studies that found being overweight or obese or having Type 2 diabetes increased the risk of dementia independently of one another.

A 2017 study published in *Diabetologia* has revealed that overweight and obese individuals with early stage Type 2 diabetes had more severe and progressive abnormalities in brain structure and cognition compared to normal-weight study participants (Yoon *et al*, 2017). The study found that grey matter was significantly thinner (atrophic) in clusters in the temporal, prefrontoparietal, motor and occipital cortices of the brains of diabetic study participants when compared to the non-diabetic control group. Further thinning of the temporal and motor cortices was also observed in the overweight/obese diabetic group, compared to normal-weight diabetics.

The effects of too much glucose (from sugars and carbohydrate foods) can create complications in the brain that accelerate cognitive dysfunction and increase the risk of dementia. The exact mechanisms of how excess glucose affects the brain is not fully understood, but insulin resistance, poor blood sugar control, and inflammation are likely to be key factors.

Our brains contain large amounts of fatty tissue – the reason for the old wives tale 'fish makes you brainy' is that the long chain polyunsaturated fats found in fish form much of the structure of the brain. However, being polyunsaturated means that these fatty acids are at greater risk of oxidative damage.

Prevention of oxidative damage is better than cure, so follow these simple dietary tips to maintain good mental health…

- Eat fish regularly (or take an omega 3 supplement)
- Include anti-oxidants to protect the long chain fatty acids – beneficial results with dementia and Alzheimer's disease have been reported with antioxidants such as vitamin E and zinc.

Meals rich in long chain fatty acids with a good helping of anti-oxidants

Breakfast Kedgeree – smoked mackerel with brown rice and wilted spinach with a small glass of orange or red grape juice

Lunch Peppered mackerel with a green leafy salad, beetroot, tomatoes, red onion and grated carrot

Dinner Tuna steak with olive oil roasted squash, sweet potato and carrots, served with broccoli.

Alzheimer's disease

Alzheimer's disease is the most frequent cause of dementia. It is caused by a build up of amyloid plaques and protein called tau, in conjunction with increased oxidative damage, causing brain cell degeneration and mental ageing. There is also thought to be a genetic factor involved, but as Alzheimer's disease has become an epidemic over the last 50 years in developed, but not undeveloped, countries, this suggests that something in the developed environment is a major risk factor, possibly exposure to excess copper or aluminium.

A 2014 systematic review searched for lifestyle risk factors for Alzheimer's disease, and concluded positive findings of ~38.9% increased risk with caffeine consumption, and 89% increased risk for lack of physical activity. Other positive links included elevated homocysteine levels, smoking, low levels of education, and low antioxidant intake. There was a protective effect from consumption of omega 3 fatty acids (Beydoun *et al*, 2014).

Nutrition to help prevent dementia and Alzheimer's disease

Fish

Research has repeatedly shown improvements in memory, cognitive performance and mental health following consumption of more omega 3 fatty acids found in fish or fish/krill oil supplements.

How does it work?

- The brain contains a high proportion of fatty tissue, of which 65% is eicosapentanoic acid (EPA) and docosahexanoic acid (DHA) – these are the long chain fatty acids found in fish.

- DHA is found in the structure of the brain, whereas EPA improves blood flow to the brain, also boosting brain function and acting as a natural anti-inflammatory. These fatty acids are essential for normal brain development and function.

- They form part of the nerve sheath that surrounds the nerve cells, maintaining membrane flexibility and providing essential insulation for electrical signals to pass from one nerve cell to another, creating our thought processes.

Docosahexaenoic acid (DHA) has been shown to be deficient in the brains of Alzheimer's patients when compared with healthy individuals of the same age, and preliminary studies indicate that low serum DHA is a significant risk factor for the development of Alzheimer's and reduced cognitive function. As fish is rich in DHA, it makes sense to include fish in our diet. Non-fish eaters could take a fish or krill oil supplement or get fatty acids from nuts and seeds such as walnuts and linseeds, which contain fats that can be converted into these longer chain fatty acids in the body. However, the conversion rate from the 'non-fish' fatty acids may be as low as 3.8% for DHA and 6% for EPA. Conversion is detrimentally affected by a diet high in saturated fats or too many omega

6 fatty acids, so if you are relying on fish-free sources of fatty acids, reduce your intake of saturated animal fats and vegetable oils or spreads rich in safflower or sunflower oil, as these foods are rich in omega 6 fats which will limit the conversion.

How much EPA or DHA do we need?

The NHS recommends eating at least two portions of fish a week, of which one portion should be oily fish. This provides approximately 450mg of omega 3 fatty acids every day; 500mg/day is generally accepted as a healthy intake. However, some people respond well to intakes of 1000mg (1g) or more daily, particularly those suffering with health conditions such as:

- Dementia

- Attention deficit hyperactivity disorder

- Depression

- Anxiety

- Autism

- Dyslexia

If you suffer with any of these health conditions and think you may benefit from more fatty acids, the first step is to adjust your diet so that you are consuming more essential fatty acids.

'To consume enough EPA/DHA, eat between one to two portions of fish each week (or up to four portions if you are not pregnant or breastfeeding), and make half of the fish you eat oily fish.'

Good sources of omega 3 fats	Fish-free options
Sardines	Linseeds or linseed oil
Salmon	Walnuts
Trout	Omega 3 fortified orange juice
Herring	Omega 3 fortified eggs
Tuna	Omega 3 fortified yoghurt
Pilchards	Green leafy vegetables

The fats found in the non-fish sources listed above are not rich in EPA or DHA, but offer the shorter chain fatty acid (alpha linolenic acid) which the body can convert into the longer chain EPA or DHA used in the brain.

Oily fish	White / non-oily fish
Salmon	Cod
Mackerel	Haddock
Trout	Coley
Herring	Plaice
Sardines	Lemon sole
Pilchards	Whiting
Tuna	Halibut
Swordfish	Skate
Kipper	Rock salmon
Anchovies	Dover sole

'Tinned fish loses much of its natural oil during the canning process, so fish such as tinned tuna and salmon will only contain approximately the same amount of omega 3 oils as fresh white fish.'

Fats for a healthy fatty acid ratio

- Reduce your intake of processed and saturated fats found in red and processed meats and confectionary foods such as cakes, biscuits, muffins and pastry

- Limit safflower or sunflower vegetable oils as these contain more omega 6 fats, which reduce conversion of the vegetable omega 3 fats into the longer chain fatty acids found in fish

- Use linseed or rapeseed oils for salad dressings as these contain more omega 3 fats and less omega 6 fats

- Use olive oil for cooking – it's not particularly rich in omega 3 fats, but contains considerably less omega 6 fats than most other oils, and is less prone to oxidation than sunflower or safflower oils. Coconut oil is an alternative for cooking based upon its limited oxidation rather than its low omega 3 content.

Omega 3-rich meal ideas

Breakfasts   Kippers and an omega 3 enriched poached egg

Kedgeree

Omega 3 fortified egg on whole meal toast

Coconut yoghurt with walnuts and linseeds

Snacks   Nut/seed bars containing linseeds/flaxseeds

A handful of walnuts

Omega 3 fortified yoghurt (dairy or soy) with added walnuts and linseeds

Lunches   Fresh (or tinned) sardines with a large green leafy salad, cherry tomatoes, beetroot and carrot

Jacket potato with tuna or salmon and salad vegetables

Seaweed, vegetable and mixed seed stir fry

Dinners   Salmon with broccoli, sweet potato and carrots

Tuna steak with roasted squash, carrots and broccoli

Spinach and sweet potato risotto drizzled with omega 3 oil and topped with walnuts.

Fruit and vegetables

Foods rich in anti-oxidants may help to prevent oxidative damage occurring, hence reducing the risk of conditions such as Alzheimer's disease. Several findings suggest that oxidative stress may play an important role in the pathogenesis of Alzheimer's, as lesions associated with exposure to free radicals are found in the brains of Alzheimer patients. There is also an increased level of antioxidants in the brain acting as free radical scavengers, and in vitro studies suggest that additional antioxidants may reduce the toxicity of amyloids in the brain. However, research findings on whether dietary or supplementary antioxidants could reduce the risk of Alzheimer's are conflicting, although there is a trend towards a positive association.

Some foods are particularly rich in phytonutrients with powerful therapeutic properties. In one study of 1836 adults, there was a reduced incidence in those who drank juices at least three times per week compared with those who drank certain types of juice less often than once per week (Dai *et al*, 2006). This was thought to be due to the polyphenol (phytonutrient) content of fruit and vegetable juices.

Eat a rainbow diet

Different coloured foods contain different nutrients. Eat a rainbow diet for maximum impact on all neurological disorders – follow the phytonutrient-rich diet in the Appendix or gain inspiration from David Heber's *'What colour is your diet?'*

Purple/red	Plums, purple grapes, strawberries, blueberries, blackberries
Red	Tomatoes, water melon, pink grapefruit
Orange	Squash, carrots, sweet potato, pumpkin, cantaloupe melon
Orange/yellow	Peaches, papaya, oranges, nectarines, apricots, tangerines
Dark green	Cabbage, broccoli, sprouts, kale, rocket, watercress
Green/yellow	Avocado, honeydew melon, peas, sweet corn, spinach
Green/white	Garlic, onions, shallots, celery, pears, chicory, chives

'Drink unsweetened red grape juice or cranberry juice every day.'

Caffeine

Current evidence linking lower incidence of Alzheimer's disease among coffee drinkers is substantial but not conclusive enough to prove a positive effect of coffee consumption on the development of this disease. There is evidence that coffee, tea, and caffeine consumption or higher plasma caffeine levels may be protective against cognitive decline and dementia. A systematic review and meta-analysis of published studies quantifying the relation between caffeine intake and dementia found a trend towards a protective effect of caffeine (Santos *et al*, 2010).

Homocysteine and the B vitamins

Homocysteine is an amino acid that occurs in the body as an intermediate in the metabolism of methionine and cysteine. Levels increase when this metabolic reaction (conversion of methionine into homocysteine, which should then be converted into cysteine) is impaired, which can be due to dietary deficiencies in vitamins B6, B9 (folic acid) or B12. As well as being an anti-oxidant, cysteine is an important protein in the body, involved in protein structure and iron, zinc and copper metabolism. If homocysteine cannot be converted into cysteine or returned to the methionine form, levels of homocysteine in the body increase.

Elevated homocysteine levels are associated with increased risk of cardiovascular disease, although some researchers suggest it may be a marker of the disease rather than a causative factor. Either way, there appears to be a link between elevated homocysteine levels and Alzheimer's disease. Zheng et al (2014) showed that plasma homocysteine concentration was higher in Alzheimer's patients with and without dementia when compared with those without Alzheimer's, concluding that hyperhomocysteine may take part in the pathogenesis of these degenerative conditions. They also found that homocysteine levels increased as duration of Alzheimer's progressed.

In addition to low levels of some B vitamins in the diet, insufficient exercise, alcohol consumption (which depletes B vitamins), high coffee consumption, smoking and some medications can all elevate homocysteine levels. A blood test for levels of homocysteine will identify your homocysteine risk, and high levels are treated with B vitamin supplementation, with advice on maintaining healthy levels with a balanced diet. One trial reported lowered homocysteine levels but no effect upon cognitive impairment or decline following supplementation with folic acid, vitamin B6, and vitamin B12 (Hankey et al, 2013), although Scott et al (2017) showed a slight improvement in cognition following B vitamin supplementation, using higher (double in most cases) amounts of B6, B9 and B12.

A double-blind controlled trial with high-dose supplementation of folic acid, vitamins B6 and B12 in individuals with mild cognitive impairment for 2 years showed the mean rate of brain atrophy (tissue loss) per year was 0.76% in the supplement group and 1.08% in the placebo group. The rate of atrophy in supplemented participants with homocysteine >13 μmol/L was 53% lower, suggesting a link between homocysteine levels and loss of brain tissue, and obvious knock on effects on cognitive function. The researchers concluded that accelerated rate of brain atrophy in the elderly with mild cognitive impairment can be slowed by treatment with homocysteine-lowering B vitamins.

Zinc

Zinc is an essential trace element that is abundantly present in the brain, playing crucial roles in learning and memory. Zinc deficiency is widespread and becomes increasingly common as we age. Zinc protects the brain from the neurotoxicity of β-amyloid protein

'A cup of coffee and of tea were included in the new graphic food pyramid designed by the National Food and Nutrition Institute in Warsaw, and American experts are of the opinion that moderate coffee intake may become an element of a proposed healthy diet.'

and it is required for many anti-oxidant enzymes, so deficiency may result in higher levels of cellular damage, including oxidative damage to brain cells. However, both depletion and excess zinc can cause severe damage to brain cells, and it is becoming more likely that a simple zinc deficiency is not the only contributor to Alzheimer's in zinc metabolism. Zinc levels in the brains of those suffering with Alzheimer's disease are often found to be considerably lower, and it has been suggested that zinc deficiency may be a significant causative factor, yet many researchers also believe that copper toxicity (often found with low zinc levels) may play a role. A recent study suggests that there may be three distinct subtypes of Alzheimer's with regard to pathophysiology, with one of them being associated with zinc deficiency. Supplementation of this mineral in Alzheimer patients has yielded positive results, but further research needs to be done.

A meta-analysis of 27 studies indicated that serum zinc appears significantly decreased in those with Alzheimer's compared with healthy controls (Ventriglia *et al*, 2015). However, in age-matched studies there was no significant difference in zinc levels between those with Alzheimer's and healthy controls, suggesting general dietary zinc deficiency with increasing age and a possible involvement of copper metabolism.

To increase your daily zinc intake...

- Add pumpkin seeds and wheat germ to cereals and yoghurts
- Eat shellfish regularly and enjoy oysters when eating out
- Eat dark cuts of meat (leg rather than breast) as they contain more zinc.

The aluminum theory

Research is inconclusive as to whether aluminium causes Alzheimer's disease, but it has been proven that as we age, blood aluminum levels increase, and those suffering with Alzheimer's disease have significantly higher levels of aluminum in their brains than normal.

The most effective way to avoid this is to limit our intake of aluminum...

- Don't use aluminum pots and pans
- Avoid using aluminium foil to wrap food
- Choose anti-perspirants that don't contain aluminium

- Avoid the use of antacids for heartburn as they contain aluminium
- Although aluminium occurs naturally in water, some water companies add it as a water treatment, so it may be worth checking with your local supplier, swapping to bottled water or using a water filter
- Don't add salt to food as aluminium is sometimes added to table salt.

Supplements to help mental function

Whilst a healthy diet is essential for good mental function, supplements can support a healthy diet and may provide a therapeutic intake if higher levels of a nutrient are beneficial. You are advised to consult a suitably qualified practitioner such as a registered nutritionist or nutritional therapist to help with supplementation.

Gingko biloba

Gingko biloba has been used as a medicinal herb for thousands of years, often used to improve memory and to help reduce the symptoms of dementia. It works by dilating (widening) the cerebral arteries and improving blood circulation to the brain. Gingko biloba contains several different active compounds including anti-oxidant flavonoids, which help to counteract oxidative damage. Although some study results have been variable, several have reported improvements in cognition with gingko biloba supplementation (Canevelli *et al*, 2014; Herrschaft *et al*, 2012).

Gingko biloba has been known to enhance:

- Memory
- Learning
- Intellect
- Emotion.

Vitamin D

Vitamin D has several associations with mental health conditions; sufficient levels are relevant for mood, ADHD, bipolar disorder, schizophrenia, and impulsive behavior due to its involvement in creating serotonin. Vitamin D supplementation may improve mood and reduce the risk of depression. A meta-analysis to estimate the association between vitamin D deficiency and risk of developing Alzheimer's disease and/or dementia was carried out in 2015. Results showed that subjects with deficient vitamin

'What we take into our body can dramatically affect our ability to stay healthy.'
Patrick Holford

D status were at increased risk of developing Alzheimer's disease by 21% compared with those with higher vitamin D levels. A significantly increased dementia risk in vitamin D deficient subjects was also found (Wong *et al*, 2015). You will increase your levels of vitamin D simply by getting a little more sunshine on the skin (without sunscreen), but some individuals may benefit from a vitamin D supplement, especially if vitamin D levels are very low, or have been low for a prolonged period of time.

B vitamins

As discussed earlier in this chapter, supplementation with B vitamins has reduced homocysteine levels and also improved some aspects of cognition. A good multi-nutrient often contains quite high levels of all B vitamins, which would be a good starting point for supplementation, rather than supplementing individual B vitamins.

Fish oils

Supplementation with omega 3 fatty acids – generally EPA and DHA – is usually 1 – 3g daily. Check the label to see how much EPA and DHA is actually in a 1g or 500mg capsule though – it is often significantly less than the 1g of fish oil. The vegetarian/ vegan equivalent of fish oil supplementation generally comes from algae, although the conversion rate (the body has to lengthen the fatty acid chain to make EPA or DHA) of the shorter fatty acids chains found in vegetables sources can be very low.

St. Johns Wort

A herb often used to improve mood is St. John's Wort, which has several medicinal uses, but is commonly taken to reduce insomnia and depression. It is thought to work through increasing the concentration or effectiveness of serotonin in the brain, enhancing a feeling of wellbeing. Research shows conflicting results and some experts state that effectiveness has not been established, although a review by Barnes *et al* (2001) stated that St John's wort appears to have a more favourable short-term safety profile than standard antidepressants. Fava *et al* (2005) compared the effects of St. John's Wort against a placebo and anti-depressant fluoxetine in a 12 week double trial with 135 patients. They found that St. John's Wort was significantly more effective than fluoxetine and showed a trend toward superiority over placebo. However, due to interaction with medicines such as warfarin, ciclosporin, theophylline, digoxin, HIV protease inhibitors, anticonvulsants, selective serotonin reuptake inhibitors, triptans and oral contraceptives, care must be taken if considering supplementation with this herb – it advised that you discuss supplementation with your doctor or a registered health practitioner.

Phosphatidyl serine

This nutrient determines the fluidity and function of cell membranes in the brain. The richest source in the diet is soya, but food does not provide enough of this nutrient, and a healthy body usually manufactures what it needs. However, if we lack essential fatty acids, folic acid or vitamin B12 in the diet, our ability to manufacture phosphatidyl serine is affected. With advancing age we seem to become less able to form this nutrient, and low levels are specifically associated with impaired mental function and dementia. Hirayama *et al* (2014) investigated whether the supplementation of soy-derived phosphatidyl serine improves ADHD symptoms in children. They found significant improvements in ADHD, short-term auditory memory, inattention and impulsivity. Moré *et al* (2014) tested 100 mg phosphatidyl serine and 80 mg phosphatidic acid on patients with Alzheimer's disease over 3 months. The researchers concluded a positive influence on memory, mood, and cognition.

Although supplementation with this nutrient may be useful, the first steps are to ensure a diet rich in the nutrients we need to naturally manufacture phosphatidyl serine in the body – fill up on these foods and see if it makes a difference to your memory!

- Eat fish, walnuts and linseeds or nut and seed oils (especially linseed oil) for the essential fatty acids you've already read so much about

- Folic acid is found in foods such as raspberries, green leafy vegetables, beans, salmon, cottage cheese and fortified breakfast cereals

- Vitamin B12 can be found in eggs, meat, fish, dairy foods, tofu and fortified cereals.

'Phosphatidyl serine supplementation has shown positive results in six double blind trials. For one participant it 'turned the (mental) clock back 12 years', giving renewed cognitive function similar to that of a 52 year old to someone aged 64!'

Please note!

Many nutrients are involved in healthy mental function, and several anti-oxidant vitamins and minerals are needed to help prevent oxidative damage that can lead to brain cell degeneration. Therefore, rather than supplement with any one nutrient, it is recommended that unless you are following a treatment plan prescribed by a qualified practitioner, a multi-vitamin, multi-mineral supplement is the best way to increase nutrient intake alongside a healthy diet. In most cases of mental impairment, best results following nutrient supplementation are observed when symptoms have been present for less than six months – when symptoms have been present for longer, it takes more time to correct nutrient deficiencies or imbalances, and in some cases the deficiencies may never fully recover, particularly in dementia and Alzheimer's disease. Even better than correcting deficiencies swiftly is preventing them in the first place: prevention is always better than cure.

Summing Up

Feeding your brain what it needs!

- Drink plenty of water to ensure adequate hydration

- Eat fish two to four times weekly for the long chain polyunsaturated fats known to benefit cognitive function

- Include foods rich in plant-based omega 3 fatty acids in your diet, such as linseeds, linseed oil, walnuts and green leafy vegetables – this is especially important if you don't eat fish

- Make sure you eat at least five servings of fresh fruit and vegetables daily to maximize your anti-oxidant intake and help prevent oxidative damage to brain cells

- Consume fruits and vegetables rich in polyphenols, anthocyanidins and anti-oxidants, in particular berries, red grapes and cherries

- Avoid sugar and refined, processed foods

- Include tryptophan-rich foods in your diet (turkey, chicken, avocado, banana, broccoli and spinach) to maximize formation of the feel good hormone serotonin

- Get plenty of sunshine so your body can make adequate amounts of vitamin D

- Try to eliminate sources of aluminium in your diet and lifestyle

- Eat a zinc-rich diet – fill up on whole grains, pumpkin seeds, seafood and lean cuts of meat

- If your diet is already good, supplementing with one or more of the nutrients discussed in this chapter may help. You are advised to seek the help of a qualified practitioner for the best supplement prescription to suit you.

A healthy digestive system

Digestive complaints are one of the most common reasons for consulting a doctor or nutritionist, and colon cancer is the fourth most common cancer in the UK, yet it is largely avoidable. Irritable bowel syndrome (IBS) is the most common diagnosis given by gastroenterologists worldwide, and over the counter remedies for heartburn and indigestion are amongst the most commonly used medications. A high fibre diet is good for our bowels, yet many people with digestive disorders cannot tolerate high fibre foods, so what then? Heartburn, indigestion and irritable bowel syndrome can all be avoided, controlled or improved through diet – which makes sense when you consider it is usually our diet causing these problems in the first place.

'Food is not classed as being in the body until it has been absorbed through the gut wall... the digestive tract creates a barrier between the exterior environment and the inside of the body.'

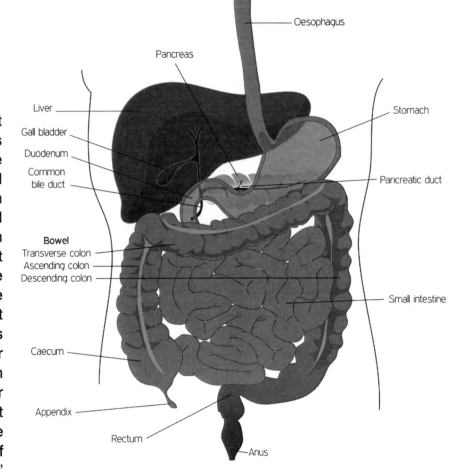

Oesophagus

Pancreas

Liver

Gall bladder

Duodenum

Common bile duct

Stomach

Pancreatic duct

Bowel
Transverse colon
Ascending colon
Descending colon

Small intestine

Caecum

Appendix

Rectum

Anus

Conditions affecting the digestive tract

Indigestion

Where indigestion is referred to as acid indigestion, this is usually the same as heartburn, but the term indigestion covers a range of symptoms including discomfort or bloating in the stomach or intestinal area.

Heartburn/acid reflux

We secrete hydrochloric acid into the stomach whenever we consume food or drinks, but various problems can occur. Heartburn can be caused by either an excess or lack of gastric acid secretion in the stomach. If too much is secreted, the food and acid mixture may travel up into the oesophagus (acid reflux), creating an uncomfortable or burning feeling. Conversely, if we don't secrete enough gastric acid, our food remains in the stomach for longer, as it fails to pass into the small intestine until it is at the correct pH and level of digestion, and this extended period in the stomach increases the risk of reflux.

The causes of acid reflux are:

- Over-secretion of gastric acid

- Under-secretion of gastric acid, delaying gastric emptying

- The lower oesophageal sphincter muscle, which usually stops acidic stomach contents from rising up into the oesophagus from the stomach, may not close properly. This may be due to physical deformity on the sphincter muscle, or hiatus hernia, or over-relaxation of the muscle, preventing it from closing completely.

A hiatus hernia is when the stomach lies higher than usual, potentially squeezing up against or through the gap in the peritoneum and diaphragm where the oesophagus normally goes. This can put pressure on the oesophageal sphincter and prevent it from closing completely. Some people are unable to completely close the oesophageal sphincter – whilst this is often a physical issue, it may also be due to dietary habits. Peppermint is commonly used to aid digestive ailments as it can relax muscles, reducing muscle spasms in the bowel. However, this property of muscle relaxation can impact on the oesophageal sphincter, over-relaxing the muscle and disabling complete closure. In a study on subjects with reflux, Jarosz and Taraszewska (2014) found an association between reflux and eating fatty, fried, sour, or spicy food and sweets, larger meals, and daily consumption of peppermint tea. Other foods and drinks commonly found to cause a problem are listed below.

Foods and drinks to avoid or reduce

- Tea and coffee

- Alcohol

- Spicy foods

- Wheat
- Dairy foods
- Citrus foods
- Eggs
- Refined carbohydrates and foods with a high sugar content
- Fatty foods
- Protein-rich meals.

Fatty foods

Fats delay gastric emptying, so as your meal remains in the stomach for longer, this can increase the risk of heartburn. Fatty meats, eggs, oily fish, cheese and other full fat dairy produce, chocolate and desserts should be avoided or limited to reduce heartburn.

Protein-rich meals

We produce acid in the stomach to kill bacteria in the food that we eat, so some gastric acid will always be secreted, even in a meal containing no protein. However, protein digestion begins in the stomach through the secretion of hydrochloric acid and enzymes, and the more protein present, the greater the amount of these secretions. Hence, if a meal is high in protein this may cause excessive acid secretion. In this case, the following foods should be limited:

- Meat
- Fish
- Eggs
- Dairy produce
- Soya products.

You may not need to eliminate these foods from your diet, but simply reduce the portion size, and the overall size of your meal, which, for most people, is a beneficial change to make anyway.

Will heartburn medicines help?

Heartburn medicine either neutralizes stomach acid, creates a barrier between the acidic stomach contents and the stomach/oesophageal mucosa, or reduces the secretion of acid into the stomach – these may alleviate your symptoms but are not removing the cause of the heartburn. Prolonged use of proton pump inhibitors that inhibit gastric acid secretion can cause a number of other issues. The acid we secrete kills microbes that we may have ingested, and reducing gastric acid secretion inhibits that antimicrobial support. There is an increased occurrence of gastrointestinal infections when proton pump inhibitors such as Omeprazole are taken, and a detrimental impact upon the entire gastrointestinal microbiome. Acid suppression has been associated with decreased absorption of dietary calcium and calcium supplements, an increased risk of hip fractures, food borne infections, and an increased risk of clostridium difficile infection (Kubo *et al*, 2014). These findings led to a recent modification in the labelling of proton pump inhibitors to include concerns about an increased risk of hip fracture. In addition to these issues, as the gastric acid is needed for protein digestion, this is compromised, and the higher pH (less acidic) in the stomach has a knock on effect to the next phase of digestion in the small intestine, affecting the secretion of bile and pancreatic digestive enzymes. This then impacts on the digestion of all nutrients consumed, and can cause additional digestive issues further on in the digestive tract. Finally, an acidic pH in the stomach is required for the absorption of several essential nutrients such as iron, calcium, magnesium, zinc, copper, iron, selenium, boron and vitamin B12. Decreased absorption of these nutrients can contribute to conditions such as anaemia and osteoporosis. So it really is better to try and figure out which foods are causing heartburn, and adjust your diet accordingly, rather than simply reduce stomach acid with medication.

'If you have heartburn, try to treat the cause, not the symptom!'

Address the cause rather than treat the symptom!

Often, gastro-intestinal secretions and function will return to normal once a food or substance that is upsetting the delicate inner lining of the gut is removed. For heartburn it may be enough to simply reduce the amount of the food culprit(s) causing problems, but sometimes it has to be removed completely. The only way to know what is causing the problem is to exclude typical or suspected foods from the diet, keep a check on your symptoms, and then re-introduce excluded foods one at a time until you can identify the food(s) causing problems. Further information on following an exclusion diet is included later on.

Lifestyle habits that increase heartburn

Certain habits and activities also increase the risk of heartburn, so adapting these may also help reduce acid reflux.

'Although it's best to figure out which foods may be causing your heartburn, and cut them out of your diet, simply avoiding lying down for a couple of hours after eating, or raising the head end of the bed on a brick can help to stop acid reflux.'

- Large meals remain in the stomach for longer, and naturally produce a higher volume of chyme (partially digested food in the stomach) – simply reducing the size of your meals is a good place to start if you suffer with reflux.

- Acidic contents have to travel against gravity up the oesophagus to cause heartburn, so leaning back, lying down or leaning over forwards all increase the risk of reflux. Avoid lounging into soft chairs or sofas after a meal, and try to eat evening meals earlier, ideally several hours before bedtime.

- If you do suffer with heartburn once retiring to bed, it can be helpful to raise your upper body so that you aren't lying flat. Try an extra pillow, or even raising the head end of the bed with a brick or some books under the bed legs.

- Activity and exercise increase the risk of acid reflux, partly because we should rest after eating and allow digestion to take place, but also the likelihood of leaning forwards and moving stomach contents around is increased. Bearing in mind that even quite simple meals can remain in the stomach for a couple of hours, and some protein-rich or fatty meals may remain for 3 – 4 hours, you may be underestimating digestion time before going out to do the gardening or some exercise.

Food and drinks that may help to alleviate heartburn

- Chamomile, fennel or ginger tea may ease heartburn with their various anti-spasmodic, anti-inflammatory properties. Some people do find peppermint tea helpful, but be mindful of consuming it too frequently as it can be a cause of heartburn as well.

- Ginger improves digestion as it activates production of saliva, gastric juice and bile, and improves gut motility.

- Bitters were traditionally taken before a meal to 'get the gastric juices flowing'. The increased secretion of gastric acid means that the stomach is prepared to receive food, and low gastric secretion is not going to delay gastric emptying and cause heartburn. Anything that stimulates digestion may work – even the smell of coffee – but bitter leaves such as rocket or dandelion, or a small piece of ginger can be used.

Undigested food and malabsorption

Apart from fibre, which passes through the gut largely undigested, all other food nutrients should be digested (broken down into smaller particles) and absorbed by the time they reach the end of the small intestine. However, in some circumstances food may not be completely digested and/or absorbed, and undigested food may even be seen in the stools. This can be as a result of:

- Food not being chewed adequately leaving food particles too large for enzymes to break them down completely

- Food passing through the gut too quickly to be thoroughly digested

- Lack of digestive enzymes, bile or other co-factors that normally aid in digestion.

If food is not being thoroughly digested and absorbed into the body, you will not be getting the nutrients and energy from food that you consume, which often results in a lack of energy and a range of symptoms linked to deficiencies in specific nutrients. Undigested food in the colon encourages 'bad' bacteria to accumulate, causing gas and putrefactive substances that alter the bowel flora and cause symptoms such as bloating and flatulence.

You may be able to recognize undigested foods in your stools, which can help you to figure out which type of foods you are having trouble digesting. For example,

- Meat fibres in the stools indicates you are not breaking down proteins

- A film of oil on the toilet water, greasy or pale coloured stools can indicate poor fat digestion

- Undigested cereal or vegetables indicates undigested carbohydrates, although remember that fibre such as tomato or pepper skins, or sweet corn outer kernels may naturally remain largely undigested.

SIBO (small intestinal bacterial overgrowth)

Most of our beneficial gut bacteria should be in the large intestine, and although certain strains of bacteria are present throughout the gut, there should not be an excessive amount in the small intestine. These bacteria feed on carbohydrate substrates – sugars, starches and fibre – and a common by product of this fermentation is hydrogen and methane gas. Whilst a certain amount of gas leaves the body via the colon, excess wind causes bloating, burping and excessive flatulence.

Causes of SIBO

- Low levels of stomach acid caused by advancing age or use of proton pump inhibitors or other medications result in higher levels of bacteria in the gut

- Gut dysbiosis, caused by antibiotics and other medications, can cause an imbalance in the gut microbiome, resulting in elevated levels of bacteria in the small intestine

- Although a high intake of sugar and/or carbohydrates is less likely to be the initial cause of SIBO, this type of diet feeds the bacteria and helps to create an ideal environment for them

- Disruption of pH (acid alkaline balance) in the gut affects the ability of the digestive enzymes to work properly, resulting in undigested food, and potentially more starches for the bacteria to feed on. Different digestive enzymes work at specific pH levels, and the small intestine should be slightly alkaline in pH, whereas gut bacteria tend to thrive in a slightly acidic environment.

The most common method of assessing SIBO is hydrogen/methane breath testing, which can be arranged by most registered nutritional therapists, nutritionists and private dieticians. Unfortunately, at the present date, SIBO breath testing is not available through the NHS. The breath test is looking for elevated levels of either methane or hydrogen to indicate bacterial overgrowth. If the test is positive, there are a number of protocols that can help address the issue.

Getting rid of SIBO

One way to kill the excess and unwanted bacteria in your gut is through a course of antibiotics prescribed by your GP. Although the NHS do not offer the SIBO breath test, if you take your results to your doctor, they may be able to prescribe a course of antibiotics to help. However, whilst this may kill the bacteria in the small intestine, it also affects the beneficial bowel flora in the large intestine, so further nutritional therapy in the form of probiotics should be considered.

Some experts suggest supplementation with probiotics in order to re-balance the microbiome as it should be, but others think that adding more bacteria to a bacterial overgrowth is not a good idea. A diet for SIBO is very low in sugar and starch, in order to starve the bacteria of their food supply. Increasing gaps between meals is also advised so there isn't a consistent supply of food for the bacteria.

It is important to discover what originally caused SIBO, otherwise the bacterial overgrowth is likely to return. A suitably qualified healthcare professional addresses overall health including the effects of medications used, digestive function, malabsorption and bowel health to find potential causes, and the resulting diet and supplement plan is individualised as required.

Helicobacter Pylori (H. pylori)

One bacterial overgrowth that can be tested through the NHS is for a bacterium called H. pylori. Infection with H. pylori creates symptoms such as heartburn and gastritis. It can be confirmed by stool, blood or breath test, or from a tissue sample taken during an endoscopy. A course of antibiotics is generally prescribed, which often eradicates the bacterial infection. However, acid-suppressing medications such as Omeprazole may also be prescribed in order to reduce gastric acid secretion, as H. pylori can infect the lining of the stomach and duodenum and cause gastric or duodenal ulcers (where the wall of the stomach or small intestine has been compromised). If an ulcer is present, the stomach or duodenum lining will be damaged by secreted acid as the underlying tissue is exposed.

FODMAP

FODMAP stands for 'fermentable oligo-, di-, mono-saccharides and polyols'. The diet originated in Australia and was been adapted for the UK by researchers. FODMAPs are sugars, sugar alcohols and short-chain carbohydrates that are poorly absorbed. They pass through the small intestine and enter the colon where they are fermented by bacteria that produce gases which stretch the bowel, causing bloating, wind and pain. FODMAPs can also cause water to move into and out of the colon, causing diarrhoea, constipation or a combination of both. FODMAPS include:

- Lactose

- Excess fructose (a sugar molecule found in fruit, sugars and vegetables)

- Types of short-chain fibres called galactans, fructans and polyols.

Studies show strong links between FODMAPs and digestive symptoms like excess gas, bloating, stomach pain and diarrhoea. Some of these substances, such as lactose, should be broken down in the digestive system and absorbed; some, like fructose, should simply be absorbed. The short chain fibres such as fructans (common in wheat, rye and barley), galactans (found in legumes) and polyols, which are in some fruits and vegetables but also in sugar alcohols like xylitol, sorbitol, maltitol and mannitol, and

'Regular use of non-steroidal anti-inflammatories can also irritate the stomach lining and cause ulcers, which is why proton pump inhibitors such as Omeprazole are prescribed with these and other drugs.'

hence found in sweeteners, are substances that wouldn't normally be digested and absorbed from the gut, but due to SIBO or some other digestive issue, more gas than usual is created from the fermentation of these substances.

For some people, these carbohydrates pass through most of the intestine unchanged, and when they reach the bowel, the bacteria that reside there feed upon these substances, creating some gas (generally methane) and short chain fatty acids. Our probiotic (good) bacteria tend to produce methane, whereas bacteria that feed on FODMAPs also produce more hydrogen gas. Excess levels of either type of gas can cause bloating, flatulence, stomach cramps, diarrhoea and constipation. Many research studies and anecdotal accounts report positive results from following a FODMAP diet; Shepherd and Gibson (2006) reported an improvement in 74% of IBS patients, and reducing foods high in FODMAPs may also be useful for people with inflammatory bowel diseases such as Crohn's disease and ulcerative colitis.

A web link with further information on FODMAPS can be found in the Appendices. However, it is not usual for individuals with IBS to be able to eat all the foods in the 'green/low FODMAP' sections and experience no digestive issues, or to have issues with all the foods in the 'red/high FODMAP' section. The usual way to use a FODMAP plan is to initially exclude all the foods high in FODMAPs for a few weeks and monitor digestive symptoms. If all of your symptoms do not improve or disappear, then there is still either an issue within the digestive system, and/or a food in the diet that you are intolerant to, and further dietary adjustment and assistance from a healthcare professional is required. However, if all symptoms abate, you can then reintroduce foods one at a time, as in a normal exclusion diet.

No gall bladder!

The gall bladder stores and squirts bile into the small intestine to help digest fats. Bile is formed in the liver, so when the gall bladder is removed, bile still travels down the common bile duct into the small intestine, but it provides a continuous trickle rather than a squirt when it is needed (when fats enter the small intestine). So if you have had your gall bladder removed, you may struggle to digest fats properly, and experience indigestion, bloating, and issues with stool formation and bowel function.

If you have had your gall bladder removed you may find it helpful to reduce fats and fatty foods in your diet, particularly:

- Cream and creamy foods
- Ice cream

- Full fat yoghurts
- Cheese, butter and margarine
- Oils
- Fatty meats
- Vegetable foods with a high fat content such as nuts, seeds and avocado.

Irritable bowel syndrome

Irritable bowel syndrome is a term used to describe a combination of gastro-intestinal symptoms such as abdominal bloating and pain, flatulence, diarrhoea and constipation, and 'dumping syndrome', when the bowel empties involuntarily. It is often worse when the individual is stressed, and can be caused or worsened by eating certain foods. Key factors usually include problems with digestion and absorption of foods, gut motility and bowel flora imbalances. The diagnosis of IBS, however, is non-specific, and often used when no obvious cause for the symptoms can be found. There are a number of potential causes for the symptoms experienced under the diagnosis of IBS.

Issues with digestion

Indigestion, bloating, abdominal discomfort and bowel issues can be caused by a number of issues:

- Reduced gastric acid secretion, poor bile flow or a lack of digestive enzymes (digestive issues)
- Food intolerances or allergies
- Disruption of the gut microflora.

Digestive issues

Bloating, discomfort, bowel issues and poor stool formation can be caused by a myriad of different things. By the time someone seeks the help of a nutritional therapist, they have usually undergone a series of tests arranged by their GP such as endoscopy or colonoscopy, and tried various medications to reduce bowel spasms, constipation or diarrhea. These may or may not have helped alleviate the symptoms, but if the medication is removed, the symptoms recur. If there are symptoms such as bloating or burping that suggest SIBO, poor digestion or malabsorption, several dietary and

'Irritable bowel syndrome is a popular medical diagnosis often reached once everything else has been excluded.'

supplement options may be considered, such as supplements or foods to enhance gastric secretion and bile flow, or digestive enzymes in the short term, until it is determined what the actual issue is.

Leaky gut syndrome

If anything irritates the gut lining, the intestinal wall can become more porous – this is known as leaky gut syndrome. Larger gaps in the intestinal cell wall allow bigger particles to move into or between the intestinal cells, often creating allergic responses as the immune system attacks these larger molecules that have not yet been fully digested. This also means that as food has not been fully broken down, you will not benefit from all the nutrients that the food has to offer. Leaky gut is often present where there is food intolerance.

Food intolerances

Food sensitivity is amongst the most common conditions that nutritional therapists are consulted for, and are often the cause of IBS symptoms. Many allergens (the substance responsible for causing a reaction) are eaten frequently and are often favorite foods; this can result in chronic, sometimes debilitating effects upon health, and due to the frequent assault on our immune system, a food allergy or intolerance can significantly reduce energy levels and affect immune function.

Whilst an allergy would stimulate antibody production in the blood (this is what skin and blood tests are looking for in food allergy tests), a sensitivity or intolerance does not necessarily create an immunological reaction that could be measured by antibodies, but there is often little difference in the symptoms experienced whether you have a sensitivity, intolerance or chronic allergy to a food or drink. Hence, the term food allergy is commonly used to refer to all three conditions, and the term 'allergen' used to refer to the offending food or drink.

Exclusion diets

There are some dietary changes that will help to alleviate a specific condition, but many recommendations will help more than one part of the gastro-intestinal (GI) tract. These changes sometimes involve removing foods from the diet that you may be intolerant of. Food intolerance can affect all parts of the digestive tract from the mouth through to the anus, so removing allergens (substances that create a reaction) may benefit the entire digestive system, and even beneficially affect other areas of the body such as the skin, mood and immune system.

Irritable bowel syndrome is often caused by one or more substances irritating the inside of the gut wall. Once this membrane is irritated, other foods that may previously have been tolerated may also cause problems. Therefore, most nutritional therapists will usually suggest an exclusion diet to identify and eradicate the food or drink culprits causing the problem. Here are some foods that are commonly excluded:

Common culprits causing IBS

- Wheat
- Gluten-containing grains (wheat, rye and barley)
- Dairy foods
- Citrus foods
- Eggs
- Chocolate
- Tea and coffee
- Alcohol

'Two thirds of IBS patients have at least one food intolerance' (Jones et al, 1982).

Sometimes, soya, spicy foods and other grains also have to be excluded, in addition to foods known to cause a problem for each individual. Wheat and dairy products are the most common culprits – Nanda et al (1989) found that 40-44% of people were intolerant to dairy and 40-60% were intolerant to grains.

The following symptoms often accompany food allergies – if you can tick two or more, you many have intolerance to something you regularly eat or drink. Whilst this list is not exhaustive, it includes many of the most common symptoms associated with a food allergy.

- Fatigue (sometimes immediately after eating a specific food, sometimes chronic fatigue, which may even be momentarily 'improved' by the allergen)
- Excess gas, flatulence, heartburn or stomach/bowel cramps
- Diarrhoea, constipation and/or poor bowel movements
- Food cravings
- Blood sugar fluctuations
- Atopic conditions (asthma, eczema, hay fever)

- Inflammatory conditions such as rheumatoid arthritis, irritable bowel syndrome or ulcerative colitis

- Moodiness, inability to concentrate, hyperactivity or depression.

Many food allergies do not produce acute reactions, and it is very common to be unaware of symptoms or fail to link symptoms to eating certain foods. A good way to identify problem foods is to keep a food diary, simultaneously noting daily symptoms. You may be able to make a link between your symptom(s) and eating a particular food; if you can't see a connection, go to see a nutritionist or dietician with your food diary.

It is common to be allergic or sensitive to more than one food at a time, and for this to be a long term problem that evades diagnosis. A food allergy may be present from birth, or it may suddenly occur during adult life. Food intolerance often develops over time, with initial reactions to a food ignored, and increased frequency of a specific allergen creating an 'adaptive' phase during which you may initially feel better for consuming it, and therefore unwittingly eat it more frequently. Finally, consuming the food or drink in question will no longer provide the 'quick fix' and temporary feeling of wellbeing, and you are left with the chronic fatigue and other symptoms that a food allergy or sensitivity can cause.

How do exclusion diets work?

Suspect foods and common allergens such as wheat and dairy foods are taken out of the diet, and re-introduced back into the diet one at a time. If symptoms improve whilst on the exclusion diet, then you have successfully removed the food causing the problems from your diet – now you need to find out which food it is! If your symptoms don't improve, then it's likely you are still eating something that is causing you problems, and may need to omit further foods from your diet.

It is essential that you consult a qualified nutritionist or dietician to help you create an exclusion diet so that you are not missing any nutrients from your diet. If one food or food group is taken out of the diet, you must ensure that the nutrients normally found in these foods are replaced by alternative foods.

How long do I have to exclude the food for?

Complete exclusion from suspect foods would normally be for at least three weeks, although some people experience an immediate change and the cause of food intolerance is identified quite quickly. Foods that have initially been excluded but are not

'If you eat two previously excluded foods together and get a reaction, you won't know which food has caused it, and will have to re-exclude both foods, and try them one at a time.'

as likely to be causing a problem can be re-introduced sooner. Sometimes allergens can never be tolerated, but often after an initial exclusion diet during which time the gut wall can mend and become fully functional, you may find that you can take small amounts of the offending food, but less frequently than before. However, if you begin to eat that food too often, the 'leaky gut' and intolerance may return, so following a rotation diet, where foods of the same 'food family' are not consumed any more regularly than once every five days, can be helpful.

Sample exclusion plan

Week 1   Take out wheat (or all gluten) products, dairy products, soya products, citrus fruits, coffee, tea, alcohol and chocolate

Week 3   Re-introduce one type of citrus fruit – if no problems occur, try another type of citrus fruit two days later

Week 4   Re-introduce another excluded item. If no symptoms re-occur, that item can remain in the diet. If symptoms return, the item is identified as an allergen and must remain excluded.

Week 5   Re-introduce another excluded food and test for symptoms. If no symptoms return, the food/drink can remain in the diet, if symptoms return, the item remains excludes.

This continues until you have a list of foods that are known to create problems and are excluded from the diet. The rest of the diet should contain a wide range of foods and not be lacking in any nutrients that the excluded food(s) contain. Sometimes the 'problem' food(s) can be re-introduced into the diet at a later stage with no problems.

Dysbiosis in the bowel

Our westernized diet rich in meat, dairy produce, sugars and refined carbohydrates and generally low in fruit and vegetables does not create a healthy bowel environment. If this describes your usual diet or you experience any of the following symptoms, which are indications of putrefactive (bad) bowel bacteria and dysbiosis (disturbed/ unhealthy bowel flora), the chances are that your bowel flora is out of balance. You can take a probiotic supplement, but this will be of little use if you continue to consume a diet that is high in sugar, refined carbohydrates and processed foods, and low in fruit and vegetables, as you are not providing the environment for the 'good' bacteria (probiotics) to thrive in.

Symptoms of dysbiosis

- Flatulence
- Diarrhoea
- Constipation
- Foul smelling stools
- Bowel cramps
- Irregular bowel movements
- Thrush
- Yeast infections such as Athlete's foot or yeast in the mouth
- Severe fatigue
- Food allergies
- Headaches.

In a healthy gut, the 'good' bacteria normally keep unhealthy organisms in check; this helps to avoid bowel conditions which can ultimately lead to irritable bowel syndrome, yeast infections such as candidiasis, ulcerative colitis, haemorroids, diverticular disease and colon cancer.

Candidiasis

Candida is a yeast organism that naturally lives in the gut. However, poor bowel conditions create exactly the right environment for our 'good' bacteria to die off, and for organisms like Candida to grow. Candidiasis can manifest as thrush, Athlete's foot, or yeast infections in the nails, mouth or stomach. Lifestyle habits that can lead to a poor bowel environment that will encourage Candida overgrowth include:

- Lots of sugar and refined carbohydrates such as white bread – Candida feeds on sugar, so eating any type of food that increases glucose levels will feed a Candida overgrowth

- Long term use of the contraceptive pill or HRT – these medications have been linked with higher incidences of thrush

- Courses of antibiotics which kill off the good bacteria as well as the bad

- Long term use of corticosteroid medication for rheumatoid arthritis, asthma or eczema – these drugs can depress immune function, making it easier for the Candida organism to grow

- Regular use of non-steroidal anti-inflammatory medication – these tablets can irritate the gut lining, increasing the likelihood of a 'leaky gut' as the gut membrane becomes more porous

- Alcohol consumption – this increases thrush as it affects glucose metabolism

- High intake of meat and dairy produce – this creates poor conditions for the 'good' bacteria in our bowel, but an ideal environment for other organisms such as Candida

- Chronic stress.

Stress has an acute effect upon the gut – it can cause decreased acid production in the stomach, leading to a more alkaline environment in which Candida thrives. Stress also suppresses immune function, making it less likely that our body will fight a Candida overgrowth.

Anything that limits the growth of healthy bacteria in the bowel will produce favorable conditions for 'bad' bacteria and fungal organisms such as Candida albicans to thrive. This imbalance in our internal flora is known as dysbiosis. There are many symptoms that might indicate Candida overgrowth – if several of these symptoms sound familiar, you may well be experiencing gut dysbiosis and/or candidiasis.

Common symptoms of candidiasis:

☐ Recurring cystitis

☐ Oral or vaginal thrush

☐ Food allergies or intolerances

☐ Food cravings, especially for sugar, bread, chocolate or alcohol

☐ Hypoglycaemia or an inability to control blood sugar levels

☐ Abdominal bloating, flatulence, heartburn and indigestion

☐ Poor bowel motility, diarrhoea or constipation, itchy rectum

☐ Fuzzy head, inability to focus, poor concentration

☐ Mood swings and depression

☐ Fungal nail infections or athletes foot

'Antibiotics kill our 'good' bacteria as well as the 'bad' bacteria, creating the ideal opportunity for Candida to thrive once our 'good' bacteria are reduced. Many women commonly experience thrush after taking antibiotics, so much so that some doctors will advise taking a probiotic when prescribing antibiotics.'

An anti-Candida diet

- Cut out sugars, alcohol and refined carbohydrates

- Limit meat and dairy foods as these contribute to more unfavourable bowel conditions

- Increase your intake of vegetables and brown rice to provide healthy fibre which creates the ideal environment for 'good bacteria' to survive in the bowel, particularly inulin-rich asparagus, Jerusalem artichoke or chicory

- Eat garlic and onion daily as these foods have anti-fungal properties and will promote the growth of 'good' bacteria in the bowel

- Limit fruit, dried fruit and fruit juice intake as these foods are a concentrated source of sugar

- Omit fermented products such as vinegar from your diet for the time being, and try to avoid foods that may harbor yeast organisms such as shelled nuts. If you do eat nuts, choose unshelled, and mushrooms are best omitted as they are a fungi and may encourage fungal growth.

- Do include fermented foods such as kefir

- Try to avoid the medications listed earlier as much as possible

- Invest in a good probiotic supplement containing Lactobacillus and Bifidobacterium species.

Diarrhoea and constipation

It is quite common to experience a combination of both diarrhoea and constipation with IBS. If the bowel is irritated by microbial infection, caffeine or other consumables, it can contract and empty the contents before the large intestine has had chance to reabsorb sufficient water – the result is diarrhoea. Although it is healthy to empty the bowel at least daily, many people in the western civilization have a bowel habit that involves emptying the bowel less frequently. Contraction of the bowel walls is controlled by the nervous system – in balance, different branches of the nervous system enable the gut to relax and contract as necessary, but factors such as stress can unbalance the nervous system and result in a tight, over-contracted bowel. Dietary factors that contribute to constipation include:

- Inadequate fluid intake

- Inadequate fibre intake.

Regular diarrhoea, constipation or inability to form and pass healthy stools may also be an indication of unbalanced bowel flora and an unfavorable bowel environment, known as dysbiosis.

Fibre

Fibre is an essential part of a healthy diet, particularly for the colon, but many IBS sufferers struggle to eat high fibre foods. However, the type of fibre makes a big difference, as some foods are rich in 'scratchy' insoluble fibre, other foods contain more soluble fibre which is much softer and kinder to the internal walls of the gastro-intestinal tract Take a look at where different types of fibre are found:

Soluble	Insoluble
Fruits	Bran and cereals containing bran
Vegetables	Whole grains (whole wheat, brown rice)
Oats and barley	Beans and pulses

Although we need both types of fibre for health, whilst the intestinal wall is irritated, you may need to limit your fibre intake to foods rich in soluble fibre, which will still help to reduce constipation and improve the bowel flora and environment. There may be occasional foods that seem to agitate your condition, but cut out as few fruits and vegetables as possible, as these are the foods containing anti-inflammatory nutrients which will ultimately improve your health.

Herbal teas to help

Peppermint, ginger or chamomile teas provide an alternative to normal coffee or tea and all have soothing properties that can help to alleviate heartburn, indigestion and IBS symptoms. However, all herbal teas should be combined with other drinks throughout the day, and in particular, don't consume peppermint tea too frequently.

The gut microbiome

Several lifestyle and dietary habits can reduce the levels of healthy bacteria in our bowel, affecting the delicate balance of flora. The most common culprits are:

- Antibiotics

- Steroids (e.g. cortisone, contraceptive pill, HRT)

- Smoking

- Stress

- Eating large amounts of meat and dairy produce, or consuming a diet high in protein

- Including large amounts of sugars and refined carbohydrates such as bread, biscuits or cakes

- Regular alcohol consumption

- Lack of dietary fibre found in fruits, vegetables and pulses.

If you can hold your hands up to more than one of these, the chances are that your bowel flora – the type of bacteria in your bowel – is not as healthy as it could be.

Bad bacteria thrive in the type of colonic environment created by high intakes of sugars, processed carbohydrates and eating too much protein food; an environment that is hostile to friendly bacteria. Once the unhealthy bacteria have grown in numbers, a battle between the 'good' and 'bad' bacteria determines which strains of bacteria inhabit the gut. The bacterial strains in the highest numbers create the colonic environment to suit their own growth and counteract further growth of any competing bacteria.

Probiotics

A good probiotic can help to re-establish the correct bowel flora, but this has to be accompanied with a good diet so that the right environment for the 'good' bacteria is created and maintained for the bacteria to survive and grow in. Probiotic supplements are likely to be much more effective than probiotic functional foods, although naturally fermented foods such as kefir do have positive effects upon the microbiome. Regular consumption of kefir has been associated with improved digestion and lactose tolerance, antibacterial effects, cholesterol-lowering effects, improved glycaemic control, anti-hypertensive effects, anti-inflammatory effects, antioxidant activity, anti-carcinogenic activity, anti-allergenic activity and healing effects, although many studies are in animal models or in vitro (Rosa *et al*, 2017). Research on the microbiome and its connections with health has grown exponentially in the past few years, and links between the gut flora and digestive disorders, allergic conditions, multiple sclerosis, Parkinson's disease, blood glucose metabolism, blood lipid health to name just a few disorders, have been proven.

'In independent tests carried out by the Food Standards Agency, some bacterial strains listed on probiotic food products such as yoghurt drinks were not even present, indicating absence at outset or that the bacteria had completely died off during production or storage.'

Supplements for digestive issues

There are many supplements that are used for digestive ailments in nutritional therapy. This is a selection of some of the most commonly used supplements.

Heartburn

A little apple cider vinegar diluted in water taken with or immediately before/after a meal may contribute to an acidic pH and aid digestion in the stomach. Deglycyrrhizinated licorice (DGL) has had the glycyrrhizin component removed to make it safer for long-term consumption. DGL may increase mucus production, which helps to coat the oesophagus and protect it from gastric acid damage, reducing the effects of acid reflux. This may be useful whilst you are adjusting your diet to remove the culprit(s) causing the acid reflux. A chewing gum developed in the USA combined DGL with other substances known to have a positive effect on acid reflux and reported a reduction in acid reflux and symptoms of heartburn (Brown *et al*, 2015), although in the UK these products are supplemented separately. Bitters supplements are also available, which stimulate gastric acid secretion.

Digestive enzymes

Taking digestive enzymes can help you to fully digest food, although you need to discover why you are not producing your own digestive enzymes, and/or why they are not effective. You can take digestive enzymes for specific types of food to break down starches, proteins or fats, or take a supplement containing a comprehensive range of digestive enzymes to aid complete digestion.

Psyllium husk

Psyllium husk is a natural soluble fibre that you add to water, juice or food. It absorbs the water it is mixed with and creates a large soft bolus which travels the length of the digestive tract to the bowel, and helps to normalize bowel function and bowel movements. Some preparations also contain probiotic 'good' bacteria. Although many studies show that psyllium fibre can reduce constipation, Attuluri *et al* (2011) found that 50g of dried prunes was more effective in their study. If psyllium husk fibre is used, it is important to increase fluid consumption too.

Slippery elm

Slippery elm formulations are typically used to help reduce inflammation in the gut. Various research studies have shown anti-inflammatory and immune modulating properties of this tree bark (Lee *et al*, 2013; Lee *et al*, 2013).

Antimicrobials

Some herbs, such as oregano, goldenseal and berberine, are natural antimicrobials and may be suggested to help with SIBO or dysbiosis (Sharifi-Rad *et al*, 2018; Arjoon *et al*, 2012).

Peppermint oil or capsules

Peppermint reduces excess or spasmodic gut contractions, so peppermint in any form can help many gastro-intestinal conditions. Peppermint oil or tea may ease upper abdominal symptoms, but for IBS or constipation, use coated peppermint capsules so that the peppermint is only released when it reaches the bowel.

Probiotics

Probiotics are commonly used to promote general good health and in conjunction with many disorders, in addition to digestive ailments. Although the strength and efficacy of the supplement is paramount, of equal importance are the strains of bacteria present, as specific strains are often used for different conditions. Didari *et al* (2015) carried out a systematic review and meta-analysis on the effects of probiotics in IBS patients. They found that probiotics reduced pain and symptom severity scores: the results demonstrated the beneficial effects of probiotics in IBS patients in comparison with placebo.

Summing Up

Although each section of the digestive tract performs a different function and has its own ideal environment, many dietary adaptations or supplements may help alleviate several different symptoms.

For improved digestion and bowel health:

- Eat plenty of fruit, vegetables and soluble fibre such as oats
- If tolerated, eat high fibre complex carbohydrates such as brown rice and pulses
- Limit sugar and refined carbohydrates
- Swap coffee and tea for anti-oxidant rich green tea or a herbal tea
- Limit alcohol intake
- Unless following a FODMAP diet, fill up on inulin-rich vegetables such as asparagus, onion, garlic and chicory for a healthy bowel
- Include linseeds for their anti-inflammatory and bowel motility benefits
- Drink approximately two litres of water each day for healthy bowel motility
- Consult a registered nutritional therapist or nutritionist to help with diagnosed digestive issues.

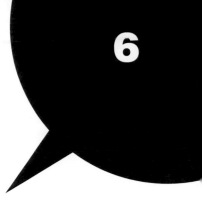

6

A diet for great skin

Our skin is made up of the compounds and nutrients from the food that we eat, so a healthy balanced diet is essential for good skin. Skin complaints such as dry, rough, itchy or flaky skin can be symptoms of dehydration or fatty acid deficiency, and may respond quickly to simple dietary changes. Eczema, dermatitis and psoriasis are common skin conditions that can respond well to nutritional medicine. With the most effective allopathic remedies such as topical steroids often causing side effects such as thinning skin, more people are searching for natural remedies to improve skin health.

Water

Water is vital for efficient metabolism and to help rid the body of toxins and waste products, and without adequate hydration, our skin can look and feel dry. An easy way to tell if you are dehydrated is by checking the colour of your urine – if it is a pale straw colour, this indicates adequate hydration.

How to increase your water intake

- Take a filled 1.5 or 2 litre bottle to work or keep it at home with you, and drink the water throughout the day – a great way to measure how much you're drinking

- Make water more interesting by infusing a jug of cool water with cucumber or lime

- Drink herbal teas or hot water with a slice of lemon or lime as a refreshing alternative to coffee or tea

- Take a small bottle of water with you when you go out in the car or on a walk so you always have something to drink

- It's essential to re-hydrate during and after exercise, as you have to replace the water that you have lost as sweat

- Fill up on foods with high water content such as melons, cucumber, tomatoes, pears and similar fruits.

'You can calculate your water requirements based upon your body weight – you need 35ml of water for every kg of bodyweight, so if you weigh 60kg, you need 35ml x 60kg = 2100ml (1.2 litres) of water daily.'

Dermatitis

Dermatitis is a term meaning inflammation of the skin, and is the same as eczema, although there are several different types.

Allergic contact dermatitis

Allergic contact dermatitis occurs when you come into contact with a substance which your body becomes sensitised to. When you touch that substance again, your skin produces an immune reaction, creating antibodies which release chemicals such as histamine. The secretion of histamine can cause an itchy red rash.

Common allergens which can trigger allergic contact dermatitis:

- Foods
- Cosmetics
- Rubber
- Some materials.
- Some metals
- Some plants
- Some topical creams.

Irritant contact dermatitis

Irritant contact dermatitis occurs when you come into contact with an irritant in detergents, soaps, perfumes, substances in toiletries or cosmetics, chemicals or some plants. As well as the usual redness, itching and inflammation, irritant contact dermatitis can cause burning, stinging and soreness, and symptoms appear immediately or within 48 hours of contact with the irritant. In either type of dermatitis, if you identify the allergens or irritants which trigger your symptoms and avoid these substances, you can reduce the frequency of flare ups.

Atopic dermatitis (commonly referred to as eczema)

This type of dermatitis has eczematous lesions, fluid-filled structures which cause characteristic weeping. If you have atopic dermatitis you are more likely to have asthma or hay fever too, and this tendency to atopic diseases is genetically inherited. People with eczema tend to have elevated IgE antibody levels and may have difficulty in fighting off certain viral, bacterial, and fungal infections, but it is often triggered by specific allergens such as soap, detergents or foods. Atopic dermatitis in particular seems to be triggered by some foods.

Nosrati et al (2017) investigated patient-reported outcomes of dietary changes upon eczema symptoms. They found that the best improvement in skin was reported when removing white flour products (53.6%), gluten (51.4%) and nightshade foods (51.4%). 79.9% of participants reported benefits from consuming more vegetables, fish oil and fruits, and the best improvement in skin was noted when adding vegetables (47.6%), organic foods (39.5%) and fish oil (35%).

Adapting your diet to counteract eczema

Tanaka et al (2001) showed that a vegetarian diet was effective for atopic dermatitis in a trial involving 20 subjects. After a two-month treatment, the severity of dermatitis was strikingly inhibited. A sharp reduction in inflammatory immune cells was observed prior to improvement in skin inflammation. Some research has shown that adjusting your intake of fatty acids may also improve eczema. Magnusson et al (2013) found that regular fish consumption in infancy reduced overall risks of allergic disease up to 12 years of age. Incidence of allergies is also reduced in offspring when fish is consumed during pregnancy. A number of foods have been linked with causing or contributing to eczema:

- Dairy foods
- Wheat and other cereals
- Eggs
- Soya products
- Caffeine
- Chocolate
- Some nuts.

'Eczema sufferers may benefit from excluding cow's milk products from the diet yet be able to consume products made with sheep or goat's milk without any detrimental effects to their skin condition.'

Excluding suspect foods

Many skin conditions, particularly eczema, respond well when allergens such as hens' eggs or dairy foods are excluded from the diet. Although many scientific trials include small numbers of people and a definitive conclusion cannot be reached about the effectiveness of exclusion diets for skin conditions, you may think it's worth a try to see if changing your diet affects your skin condition.

A number of foods can all be excluded on the same diet – exclude them all in one go at the start then bring them back in to your diet one at a time to test them. It will help to keep a note of which foods you try and the reactions that you experience – this will enable you to create a list of foods that you know you can eat, and a list of foods to avoid if they worsen your eczema. Try to stay on the exclusion diet for inflammatory skin conditions in the Appendices for at least three weeks, and then if symptoms have improved, either continue with the diet, or try to re-introduce one food at a time in order of the foods you think are least likely to cause a problem. This way, you'll be able to widen the variety of foods in your diet more quickly.

Here's an example of a list of initially excluded foods that could be reintroduced back in to the diet one at a time. Foods or drinks that cause no problems or skin flare ups are left in the diet once re-introduced, but anything that worsens or causes symptoms is taken back out of the diet.

Foods to try	Date tried	Comments
Coffee with no milk		
Bread		
Eggs		
Sheep or goat yoghurt		
Sheep or goat's milk		
Cow's milk yoghurt		

Adjusting your fatty acid intake

As well as following an exclusion diet, an anti-inflammatory diet is also recommended as eczema is an inflammatory skin condition. Adjusting the ratio of fatty acids by increasing the amount of omega 3 fats whilst reducing the amount of omega 6 fats is particularly recommended. In 2008, Koch *et al.* tested the effects of docosahexaenoic acid (a type of omega 3 fish oil) on eczema patients and concluded that 'DHA could be bioactive and might have a beneficial impact on the outcome of atopic eczema', although greater numbers are needed for more conclusive research. Vegetarian diets have also shown positive results on inflammatory skin disorders. Although some research shows positive effects on eczema following supplementation with evening primrose oil, a review of 27 trials concluded that the effect of borage oil and evening primrose oil was no better than placebo (Bamford *et al*, 2013).

How to eat more fats with anti-inflammatory properties

- Eat more oily fish such as tuna, salmon, pilchards, mackerel, sardines

- Tinned fish and white fish such as cod, haddock and plaice also contain omega 3 fats, although not as much as the oily fish

- Reduce the amount of meat you consume as this contains more arachidonic acid, which increases pro-inflammatory mediators

- Linseeds and walnuts are rich sources of alpha-linolenic acid, which the body can convert into the longer chain fats found in fish

- Don't use safflower or sunflower vegetable oils as these contain more omega 6 fats which limit the conversion of the vegetable omega 3 fats into longer chain fatty acids

- Use linseed or rapeseed oil for salad dressings as these oils have a good omega 3: omega 6 ratio.

Tea drinking may have therapeutic effects

Some research indicates that the polyphenols found in tea may have beneficial effects upon skin conditions. One study found that 63% of patients who drank one litre of Oolong tea each day (three equal servings after each meal) showed marked to moderate improvement within one month of treatment (Uehara *et al*, 2001). Green (and black) tea also contains therapeutic nutrients with anti-inflammatory properties.

Zinc

Zinc deficiency is common in acne and eczema sufferers, and plays a major role in skin health and immune function. Zinc is found in meats (particularly the dark cuts of meat), oysters, offal, whole grains, pumpkin seeds, asparagus and watercress. Kim *et al* (2014) showed that hair zinc levels in children with atopic dermatitis were lower than in controls without eczema, and supplementation with zinc improved pruritus. If you think it's going to be difficult to increase your zinc intake (for example if you are vegetarian), take a multi-mineral containing at least 15mg of zinc.

Psoriasis

The prevalence of psoriasis in Western populations is estimated to be around 2 – 3%, and despite several different types of treatment including orthodox medicines, phototherapy (treatment with sunlight/UV light) and ichthyotherapy, where doctor fish eat the psoriatic plaques, there appears be no actual cure.

The cause of psoriasis is still unknown; although there appears to be a genetic tendency and an irregularity in immune regulation. Psoriasis is characterised by red, scaly patches on the skin, caused by excessive skin production and inflammation. It normally takes approximately one month for skin cells in the epidermis to gradually become keratinised and move to form the outer layer of skin, but this process is accelerated in psoriasis, creating too much skin which pushes together forming crusts and plaques.

Certain foods may trigger flare ups of psoriasis, and factors that also aggravate psoriasis include:

- Stress
- Alcohol
- Smoking
- Withdrawal of systemic corticosteroids.

Finding ways to manage stress more effectively, stopping smoking and reducing alcohol intake may help to reduce or manage psoriasis. In addition to these lifestyle adjustments, there are a number of dietary changes that you can try. Fasting, vegetarian diets, and diets rich in omega-3 fatty acids from fish oil have all been associated with improvement in some studies, but conclusive evidence on the efficacy for treating psoriasis with any of these dietary interventions is lacking. However, an anti-inflammatory diet designed to support immune function will be therapeutic for overall health and may help to reduce the severity of psoriasis.

Adapting your diet to counteract psoriasis

There are several elements to consider in a therapeutic diet for psoriasis. Ideally, you need to:

- Support immune function with anti-oxidants

- Follow an anti-inflammatory diet as this is an inflammatory skin disease

- Consider following an exclusion diet to encourage optimal intestinal and bowel function – this will also support liver function and natural detoxification pathways, easing the workload on the immune system

- Avoid foods that may trigger flare ups of psoriasis

- Ensure a rich source of certain vitamins and minerals in the diet.

Although this may seem like lots of different dietary adjustments, most of these changes are helpful in more than one way. For example, anti-oxidants such as Vitamin E and selenium are also anti-inflammatory and will support liver function, and the foods rich in anti-oxidants are also those that support healthy intestinal and bowel function.

Support immune function with anti-oxidants

If you have psoriasis it can be beneficial to eat a diet rich in anti-oxidants such as vitamins C and E, selenium, zinc and beta carotene. These nutrients are helpful in most skin conditions, so tips on how to eat more zinc, beta carotene and vitamin E can be found in the sections on eczema and acne.

Vitamin C

Vitamin C has anti-inflammatory properties, so any inflammatory skin condition may benefit from therapeutic doses of this vitamin. Both vitamin C and vitamin E also support and help to normalise immune function. Foods rich in vitamin C include citrus fruits, berries, green leafy vegetables, peppers, kiwi fruit and potatoes.

How to increase your dietary intake of vitamin C

- Add berries and kiwi to yoghurt or breakfast cereals
- Add rocket to pasta and rice dishes
- Add watercress or spinach to salads and sandwiches.

Selenium

'It's better to place potatoes directly into boiling water as they lose much of their vitamin C content in the first two minutes of cooking.'

As well as being an important anti-inflammatory and anti-oxidant, selenium is required for detoxification processes, so it helps to reduce toxin levels in the skin. It works synergistically with vitamin E, so it's a good idea to take these two anti-oxidants together. Foods rich in selenium include Brazil nuts, sunflower seeds, whole grain cereals, seafood and offal.

How to increase your dietary intake of selenium

- Snack on nuts, particularly Brazil nuts
- Enjoy a prawn sandwich or crab salad for lunch
- Increase seafood intake with paella or scallops.

Eat an anti-inflammatory diet

An increased intake of omega 3 fatty acids has improved psoriasis in some trials, probably as a result of reduced pro-inflammatory arachidonic acid intake, and increased anti-inflammatory eicosapentaenoic and/or docohexanoic acids from fish intake, resulting in an overall anti-inflammatory effect.

Due to the inflammatory nature of skin conditions, it makes sense to fill up on foods such as green leafy vegetables, fish, walnuts and linseeds, which all contain nutrients with anti-inflammatory properties:

Ways to increase your anti-inflammatory fatty acid intake

- Swap meat for fresh or tinned fish in sandwiches
- Swap cured meats to sardines on toast
- Swap bacon and eggs to kedgeree or kippers
- Swap roast meats at dinner for salmon or tuna steak
- Use tuna or soya mince in place of mince in pasta dishes
- Add linseeds and walnuts to cereals, yoghurts, salads and stir fries
- Try bars with added seeds such as the '9 bar' with linseeds
- Snack on walnuts
- Add onion and rocket, watercress or spinach to sandwiches and salads
- Add rocket to rice and pasta dishes
- Eat onions every day – add to sandwiches, salads, omelettes and base each cooked meal on onions.

Try an exclusion diet

There are several reasons to find an exclusion diet that suits you if you suffer with psoriasis. Research has shown a correlation between psoriasis and dysfunction in the digestive tract and bowel, with significant links between gluten intolerance and psoriasis. Studies also show potential links between arthritis and gout occurring with psoriasis, both of which flare up with specific foods.

Links between psoriasis and gluten intolerance

Patients with psoriasis have a higher prevalence of other autoimmune diseases including coeliac disease (severe gluten intolerance). Several studies have illustrated links between psoriasis and dysfunctional digestion or poor bowel health, providing evidence that a gluten free diet can improve the condition (De Bastiani et al, 2015). To avoid gluten you must exclude all products made with wheat, rye and barley, consuming no bread, pasta, cous cous, biscuits or cakes unless they are made with gluten free flour. If you want to try a few days to see how your psoriasis reacts, try the gluten free eating plan in the Appendices.

Links with arthritis or gout

According to the USA National Psoriasis Foundation, studies show that between 10 and 30 percent of people with psoriasis also develop psoriatic arthritis. There may be links between the development of rheumatoid arthritis or gout and psoriasis, indicating that dietary adaptations that suit these conditions may also benefit psoriasis.

Gout is likely to be caused by foods that are rich in purines, and exacerbated by foods that increase urate salt production, so it may be worth reducing these foods in your diet:

- Game, meat and offal
- Herrings, sardines, shellfish and fish roe
- Sugars and refined carbohydrates
- Fruit
- Yeast
- Alcohol

Avoid trigger foods

Most of these so called 'trigger foods' are not included in a healthy exclusion diet, however, your 'trigger' foods may be different to someone else's, so exclude any foods that seem to cause a flare up in symptoms, but include any healthy foods from this list that don't cause a problem... there's little point including cola drinks or mono-sodium glutamate as they won't benefit your overall health, but tomatoes and berries contain important nutrients known to benefit health, so you should eat them if you can.

Most likely trigger foods for psoriasis:

- Red meat
- Refined carbohydrates and bakery goods – white bread, cakes, biscuits etc.
- Cola
- Red wine (and alcohol generally)
- Mono-sodium glutamate (an additive often found in Chinese take-away and savoury snacks)
- Chili and other hot spices

- Berries
- Tomatoes

Vitamin D

We make vitamin D in the skin when we expose our skin to the sunlight, and as psoriasis often improves in the sun, large pharmacological doses of Vitamin D have been used in dermatology for the treatment of psoriasis. The active form of vitamin D exhibits anti-proliferative and immune regulating effects, and has been shown to be useful in the treatment of psoriasis. Soleymani *et al* (2015) found that oral and topical vitamin D therapies provide comparable efficacy to corticosteroids when used as mono-therapy and may be superior when used in combination with a topical steroid. However, Mercola *et al* (2014) investigated the association between dietary, supplementary and total vitamin D intake and the incidence of psoriasis in 70,437 women. They found no significant association between vitamin D intake (dietary, supplementary and total vitamin D) and the incidence of psoriasis and concluded that vitamin D seemed to have no preventative or treatment role for psoriasis.

Ways to get more vitamin D in your diet

- Oily fish
- Eggs
- Butter
- Liver
- Margarines and cereals fortified with vitamin D

However, as some of these foods may be excluded from a therapeutic diet for psoriasis, you may want to top up vitamin D levels with a little sunshine and a good multi-vitamin supplement containing vitamin D.

'Optimum nutrition is different for everyone.'

Acne

Acne is characterized by inflammatory and non-inflammatory spots and pimples caused by hair follicles blocked with plugs of sebum and dead skin cells. Production of sebum from the sebaceous glands in the skin is affected by secretion of androgen (sex) hormones, and there is a link between higher testosterone levels and acne (in females and males).

Things that increase the risk of acne:

- Family history

- Increased/altered hormonal activity, for example, during puberty or menopause, or as a result of taking anabolic steroids

- Hormonal changes due to other medical conditions such as polycystic ovarian syndrome

- Over secretion of sebum, usually linked to hormone (testosterone) levels.

However, although sebum excretion is influenced largely by genetic factors, environmental factors do contribute to the risk of developing acne. Stress also makes acne worse, and there are a number of links between diet and acne. In their 2009 review, Spencer *et al* found that acne prevalence is lower in rural societies than in westernized populations. Several researchers have reported that remote islanders eating mainly root vegetables, fruit, fish, and coconut, with minimal intake of dairy products, coffee, alcohol, cereals, oils, sugar, and salt have no acne.

Dietary habits that may cause or contribute to acne:

- High GI carbohydrates such as cakes, biscuits and white flour products

- Milk and other dairy products in the diet

- Low intakes of vitamins A and E.

Adapting your diet to counteract acne

Although there has been a long held assumption that a 'junk food' diet causes acne, more research in this area has identified more specific food groups that appear to contribute to this skin condition. In fact, research states that the effects of chocolate on acne are 'inconclusive' as it neither improved nor worsened the condition, unlike high GI carbohydrate foods. An 'anti-acne' diet is a Palaeolithic-like diet with reduced intake of sugar, grains, milk and milk products, but including plenty of vegetables and fish.

Avoid high GI carbohydrates

Carbohydrates which cause high glucose levels and stimulate insulin secretion have been linked with acne (Mahmood and Bowe, 2014). Insulin triggers the release of insulin-like growth factor (IGF), which in turn, affects the sebaceous glands, skin secretion and metabolism. Insulin resistance causing elevated blood glucose and high insulin levels is found in polycystic ovarian syndrome, where acne is a common complaint.

Smith *et al* (2007) compared the results of a low glycemic diet with a high glycemic diet on clinical and endocrine aspects of acne vulgaris. After 12 weeks the total lesion counts had decreased more in the experimental group (low GI diet) compared with the control group (high GI diet). Burris *et al* (2017) also found that those with worse acne consumed more carbohydrate foods, and had greater insulin, insulin-like growth factor-1 concentrations, greater insulin resistance, and lower sex hormone-binding globulin concentrations compared to participants without acne. These are all factors that are linked with the occurrence of acne, and confirm a relationship between dietary carbohydrate, overall glycaemic load and acne.

To change your diet to a low GI diet:

- Swap white bread for rye, pumpernickel or whole meal bread
- Exclude biscuits, muffins, pastries and cakes from your diet, swapping these foods for oat or nut-based snacks
- Eat fruit instead of sweets
- Follow a reduced sugar, reduced carbohydrate, paleo-type diet.

Dairy and acne

There appears to be a link between consumption of milk and other dairy products and acne, although some researchers suggest this may be due to the effects of hormones in the dairy produce rather than the food itself. Melnik (2009) suggests that consumption of cow's milk and cow's milk protein results in changes between insulin, growth hormone and insulin-like growth factor-1 in humans, raising IGF-1 serum levels. IGF-1 serum levels are particularly high during puberty, and are further enhanced by milk consumption, explaining the correlation between milk consumption and acne in teenagers. Several other research studies have found a positive association between acne and milk intake (Ismail *et al*, 2012; Adebamowo *et al*, 2006). With this amount of evidence suggesting a link between cow's milk and acne, if you suffer with this skin condition it is worth excluding dairy – at least cow's milk products – from your diet. There are plenty of non-dairy alternatives available, including coconut, nut, soya, oat or rice milks.

Vitamins A, vitamin E and zinc (anti-oxidants)

Studies have shown that newly diagnosed acne patients sometimes have lower levels of vitamin A, vitamin E and zinc. Adequate amounts of vitamin A naturally inhibit sebum secretion from the sebaceous glands, and many acne medications are based upon vitamin A (retinol) therapy, although these have a number of side effects, and when treatment finishes the acne often reappears. As well as having an anti-inflammatory role in acne control, Vitamin A reduces the creation of acne lesions by reducing clogged pores and modifying how dead skin cells are removed.

Ozuguz *et al* (2014) evaluated plasma levels of vitamin A, E and zinc in acne patients, and found that levels of vitamin E, vitamin A and zinc were significantly lower in those with acne. In addition, levels of vitamin E and zinc were even lower in those with severe rather than mild acne, illustrating a negative correlation between acne severity and vitamin E and zinc levels. Another study evaluated the effects of supplementing vitamin E and zinc combined with lactoferrin, an iron-binding milk-derived protein that has antibacterial and anti-inflammatory effects. It significantly reduced acne lesions in people with mild to moderate acne vulgaris (Chan *et al*, 2017).

To help prevent, or improve, acne through diet, look for a rich source of these anti-oxidants. Food sources of vitamin A include milk, cheese, eggs, and beef or chicken liver. However, as dairy foods may possibly increase the risk of acne, vegetable sources of beta carotene are a good way to boost your vitamin A intake. Beta carotene has pro-vitamin A activity, meaning that it can be converted into vitamin A as and when required, and any excess beta carotene is largely removed in urine. Beta-carotene has also been proven to offer skin protection to sun exposure to the extent that taking beta-carotene supplements before sun exposure has been widely recommended.

Foods and meals rich in beta carotene

Sweet potato, carrots, squash, pumpkin, mango, papaya, apricots, green leafy vegetables and beetroot.

Breakfast Blend cantaloupe melon and peaches with soy yoghurt or banana and a little linseed or rapeseed oil for a beta-carotene smoothie

Lunch   Corn tortilla wrap with spinach, avocado, peppers, grated carrots, tomatoes, beetroot and pumpkin seeds

Dinner   Salmon with asparagus, roasted carrots and sweet potato

Snacks   Apricots, mangoes, peaches, nectarines

Heavy cooking can destroy much of the beta carotene in vegetables, but light cooking, mashing or puréeing may enhance its availability and absorption as the plant cell walls are ruptured and open up to release the beta carotene within. It is best absorbed with some fat in the meal, so combine orange fruits with seeds or nuts, and roast pumpkin, sweet potato or carrots with a little olive oil to enhance absorption, providing vitamin E at the same time.

Vitamin E

Vitamin E provides multiple benefits for skin health, as it provides anti-oxidant, anti-inflammatory and immune-supportive properties.

- It supports immune function which is over-stimulated in eczema, dermatitis and acne
- It reduces free radical damage, which is a significant cause of 'ageing', which is why it's found in so many face and body creams.

Foods rich in vitamin E include vegetable oils, nuts (especially almonds, Brazils and hazelnuts), pine nuts, sunflower seeds, avocado and wheat germ.

How to increase your dietary intake of vitamin E

- By snacking on nuts and seeds
- By drizzling high quality, cold vegetable oils on to salads
- By adding pine nuts to salads and stir fries
- By adding wheat germ to cereals or yoghurts
- By adding avocado to salad sandwiches, salads and wraps.

Supplements to help skin conditions

Fatty acids for eczema

If you don't eat much fish it can be difficult to consume enough omega 3 fatty acids, especially as the conversion rate from vegetable sources of walnuts or linseeds can be low. Therefore, a fatty acid supplement may be helpful – look for EPA and DHA, and take 1g of EPA and DHA (1000mg) daily.

Probiotics for all skin conditions

In their review, Schlichte *et al.* (2016) reported promising results on atopic dermatitis with the use of probiotics and prebiotics taken in combination. Probiotics have been reported to prevent atopic sensitisation to common food allergens, reducing the incidence of atopic eczema in early childhood. Mansfield *et al* (2014) analysed the impact of prenatal and postnatal probiotic supplementation on the prevention of childhood eczema, and concluded that the use of probiotic supplements during pregnancy and/or during infancy creates a statistically significant decline in the incidence of eczema. Some studies show disturbed skin flora and also differences in bacterial ratios in the gut microbiome in those with psoriasis, and several trials show benefits in acne, eczema and psoriasis following probiotic supplementation (Notay *et al*, 2017).

Vitamins A, E and zinc for acne

Studies have shown that levels of these nutrients are often lower in those with acne, so supplementing with vitamin A (or beta carotene), vitamin E and zinc may be beneficial.

Summing Up

There are a number of nutrients required for healthy skin, and creating a healthy diet based upon these elements will improve the overall condition of skin, as well as improve many skin conditions.

- Eat the right ratio of fatty acids – more omega 3, less omega 6
- Excluding common allergens such as dairy or gluten may help
- Include lots of anti-oxidant rich foods to reduce inflammation and promote healthy skin formation and function
- Eat low GI carbohydrates and cut down on refined carbohydrates
- Drink plenty of water – up to two litres every day.

Stick to…	Stay away from…
Lots of water	Food allergens that may exacerbate your skin condition
Low GI carbohydrates	Sugars and refined, high GI carbohydrates
Anti-oxidant rich foods packed with vitamins A, C, E, zinc and selenium	
Omega 3 rich foods – fish, linseeds, walnuts	

Appendix A

Therapeutic eating plans

Therapeutic diet for hypertension and atherosclerosis

Monday	Porridge made with water/soya milk, mixed seeds and fruit
Mid-morning	Homemade hummus (chickpeas, olive oil, garlic) with celery, raw asparagus and radish
Lunch	Tomato soup and two oatcakes
Dinner	Baked salmon steak with broccoli, cauliflower and baked sweet potato
Tuesday	Soya or coconut yoghurt with flaked almonds and cherries
Mid-morning	Celery and pepper crudités
Lunch	Mixed bean and brown rice salad with tomatoes, garlic, onions, cucumber, radish and chicory, a sprinkle of olive oil
Dinner	Seared tuna steak with roast potatoes, parsnips, carrots and broccoli
Wednesday	Granola (toasted oats and seeds) mixed with oats and fruit
Mid-morning	A handful of almonds or olives
Lunch	Sardines with chicory, onion, garlic, asparagus, celery and beetroot
Dinner	Savoy cabbage/red onion/garlic stir fry with 50g brown rice
Thursday	Porridge with water/soya milk, almonds, linseeds and fruit
Mid-morning	Oatcakes with hummus, celery, raw peppers and carrot
Lunch	Peppered mackerel with a large mixed salad with chicory
Dinner	Stuffed peppers and potatoes with a large green salad
Friday	Fruit salad sprinkled with mixed nuts and seeds
Mid-morning	A handful of nuts or olives
Lunch	Omelette with tomatoes, rocket and mushrooms, with salad
Dinner	Bean, tofu and vegetable curry, chill or stew with brown rice
Saturday	Banana and egg pancakes with yoghurt and nuts/seeds
Snacks	Celery, peppers and carrot crudités with hummus
Lunch	Tomato and lentil soup
Dinner	Steamed fish with potatoes, carrots and asparagus

Sunday	Kedgeree made with mackerel, brown rice, onion and garlic
Mid-morning	A few nuts or olives
Lunch	Roast dinner with plenty of vegetables and low salt gravy
Dinner	Watercress or broccoli soup with oatcakes

... and maybe an occasional glass of red wine if you're having a tipple!

Therapeutic exclusion diet for rheumatoid arthritis or osteoarthritis

Monday	Porridge with soya milk and added walnuts and seeds
Mid-morning	Piece of fruit – apple, pear, apricot or peach
Lunch	Watercress soup with oatcakes
Dinner	Seared tuna steak with broccoli, cauliflower and roasted squash

Tuesday	Millet/oat flakes with soy yoghurt, walnuts and linseeds
Mid-morning	Raw carrot and cucumber crudités with hummus
Lunch	Corn tortilla wrap with salad – rocket, cucumber, radish, celery and avocado with added walnuts and linseed oil
Dinner	Baked salmon steak with carrots, broccoli and baked sweet potato

Wednesday	Spinach and banana smoothie made with water
Mid-morning	Handful of walnuts or olives
Lunch	Mixed bean and rice salad with vegetables
Dinner	Savoy cabbage/red onion/garlic stir fry with rice noodles

Thursday	Porridge with soya milk, fruit, linseeds and nuts
Mid-morning	Cherries and/or red grapes with soy yoghurt
Lunch	Sardines with a large green salad, beetroot, carrot and onion
Dinner	Brown rice and tofu vegetable risotto

Friday	Granola (toasted oats and mixed seeds) with soya milk
Mid-morning	Celery, mange tout and carrot
Lunch	Poached egg with asparagus
Dinner	Mixed bean and vegetable curry or chill and brown rice

Saturday	Oat/millet flake porridge with soya milk and added linseeds
Snacks	Raw vegetables or fruit
Lunch	Home made vegetable soup with oatcakes
Dinner	Steamed lemon sole or trout with peas, cabbage and squash

Sunday	Kippers and a poached egg with spinach
Mid-morning	A piece of fruit
Lunch	Roast dinner with plenty of vegetables but little/no meat
Dinner	Watercress or broccoli soup with oatcakes

... and add anti-inflammatory turmeric or ginger to foods every day!

Therapeutic diet for osteoporosis

Monday	Porridge made with soya milk, mixed nuts and seeds
Mid-morning	Handful of mixed nuts – almonds, walnuts, cashews, pecans
Lunch	Tomato and lentil soup (with gluten-free oat cakes if desired)
Dinner	Baked salmon steak with carrots, broccoli and baked sweet potato

Tuesday	Gluten-free muesli and soy yoghurt with flaked almonds
Mid-morning	Raw carrot and pepper crudités dipped in hummus
Lunch	Tinned sardines on wholewheat toast, rocket and beetroot
Dinner	Seared tuna steak with broccoli, cauliflower and baked sweet potato

Wednesday	Porridge with soya milk, flaked almonds and mixed fruit
Mid-morning	Raw vegetables (asparagus, tomatoes, olives) with hummus
Lunch	Mixed bean and chickpea salad with peppers, tomatoes, olives, rocket and onions
Dinner	Savoy cabbage or kale/red onion/garlic/vegetable stir fry with seeds or pine nuts. Lean beef or chicken can be added.

Thursday	Soya yoghurt with plums, cherries and flaked almonds, pumpkin seeds
Mid-morning	Handful of nuts or dried soya beans
Lunch	Peppered or fresh mackerel with a large green salad, beetroot, carrot, red onion, cucumber and radish
Dinner	Brown rice (50g) vegetable, chicken or salmon risotto

Friday	Banana (1), egg (2) and ground almond pancakes – mix into a batter and lightly fry small pancakes
Mid-morning	Oat/corn cakes with homemade hummus, celery, raw peppers and carrot
Lunch	Jacket potato with baked beans or hummus, and a mixed salad
Dinner	Mixed bean and vegetable curry or chilli with steamed brown rice

Saturday	Poached eggs on a bed of spinach
Snacks	Oatcakes with sliced banana
Lunch	Mung bean or lentil and vegetable soup
Dinner	Steamed lemon sole or trout with vegetables and potatoes

Sunday	Kedgeree or kippers with a poached egg
Mid-morning	A handful of cherries or couple of plums, or a handful of nuts
Lunch	Roast Sunday dinner with plenty of vegetables
Dinner	Sardines or mackerel with a large green salad, tomatoes, olives, grated carrot, beetroot and peppers, pine nuts.

... and don't add any salt!

Therapeutic diet for diabetes and insulin resistance

Monday	35g porridge made with soya milk and cinnamon, mixed seeds or nuts and berries
Mid-morning	Piece of fruit – apple, kiwi or cherries
Lunch	Tomato and lentil soup with1 slide pumpernickel, rye or sourdough bread
Dinner	Baked salmon steak with avocado and large mixed salad

Tuesday	Coconut or live sheep/goat yoghurt, flaked almonds, cherries
Mid-morning	Celery or pepper crudités
Lunch	Mixed bean or tuna salad with tomatoes, onions, cucumber, radish, celery, avocado
Dinner	Brown rice (50g) vegetable risotto with garlic and onion

Wednesday	35g porridge with soya or skimmed milk, cinnamon and berries or cherries
Mid-morning	Cherry tomatoes, baby corn, cucumber, carrot
Lunch	Sardines with a large green salad, onion, garlic, carrots, tomatoes and beetroot
Dinner	Savoy cabbage/red onion/garlic/mushroom stir fry with other vegetables

Thursday	Poached egg with asparagus
Mid-morning	Raw peppers, raw carrot and celery crudités
Lunch	Peppered mackerel salad with avocado, asparagus, tomato, watercress and beetroot
Dinner	Roast chicken/turkey or salmon/tuna with stir-fry vegetables

Friday	Soy or live yoghurt with mixed seeds and berries or cherries
Mid-morning	Piece of fruit or piece of cooked chicken, turkey or mackerel
Lunch	Small baked potato with tuna and a mixed salad
Dinner	Smoked fish salad with avocado, cucumber, rocket, celery, tomatoes, beetroot

Saturday	35g porridge with soya milk, cinnamon and berries/cherries
Snacks	Tomatoes, raw peppers and carrot crudités
Lunch	2 egg omelette with mushrooms, onion, spinach, tomatoes and a little cheese with salad
Dinner	Steamed fish with broccoli and garlic roast parsnips, carrots and sweet potato

Sunday	Banana and egg pancakes
Mid-morning	Handful of nuts or a few olives
Lunch	Roast Sunday dinner (no/limited potatoes)
Dinner	Watercress soup and oatcakes

... and drink green tea!

Therapeutic diet to improve mood and cognitive function

Monday	Porridge with soya milk with walnuts and raspberries
Mid-morning	Celery, tomato, carrot and radish crudités
Lunch	Peppered mackerel with a green leafy salad, beetroot, tomatoes, red onion and grated carrot and seeded bread
Dinner	Spicy bean chili with brown rice
Tuesday	Fruit salad with mixed berries, mango, apricots, peach, kiwi and red grapes with soy or live yoghurt and mixed seeds
Mid-morning	Carrot and pepper crudités
Lunch	Mixed bean salad with chick peas, tomatoes, garlic, onions, cucumber, radish and walnuts
Dinner	Stir fried tofu with onion, mushroom, peppers, peas, corn
Wednesday	Scrambled egg with rocket, tomatoes, red onion and mushrooms on pumpernickel bread
Mid-morning	Nut/seed bar or handful of red grapes
Lunch	Sardines on whole meal toast with a dark green leafy salad
Dinner	Savoy cabbage/red onion stir fry with baby corn, tofu, mange tout, sesame and fenugreek seeds or pine nuts
Thursday	Omega 3 fortified boiled egg with toasted whole meal bread
Mid-morning	Handful of nuts or a plum
Lunch	Lentil soup and oatcakes
Dinner	Salmon and sweet potato risotto with rocket or spinach
Friday	Soy yoghurt with sliced kiwi, cherries, raspberries, flaked almonds and pumpkin seed mix
Mid-morning	Tomatoes, raw peppers and carrot crudités with hummus
Lunch	Corn tortilla wrap with turkey, bean sprouts, rocket, tomatoes
Dinner	Tuna steak with olive oil roasted squash, sweet potato and carrots, served with broccoli

Saturday	Poached omega 3 fortified egg on whole meal toast
Snacks	A handful of cherries
Lunch	Lentil soup and oatcakes
Dinner	Baked fish/organic meat with roast vegetables and cabbage
Sunday	Kedgeree or kippers, poached egg and spinach
Mid-morning	Coconut yoghurt with kiwi, orange segments and pumpkin seeds
Lunch	Roast dinner
Tea	Salmon and avocado on toasted seed bread with green leaf and walnut salad, linseed dressing juice.

Therapeutic diet for SIBO

Monday	Poached eggs on a bed of spinach
Lunch	Chicken/turkey or fish homemade soup
Dinner	Baked salmon steak with Chinese stir fry: bok choy, bamboo shoots, ginger and other spices/herbs allowed – no sauce
Tuesday	Lactose free yoghurt with nuts (almonds, pecans, brazils, hazelnuts, walnuts, cashews, chestnuts)
Lunch	Fish or meat with raw carrot, bean sprouts, celery, lettuce, olives, spinach, tomatoes
Dinner	Seared tuna or beef steak with green beans, braised lettuce (not chicory/endive) and roasted/baked red peppers
Wednesday	Egg and banana pancake (use brown banana)
Lunch	Sardines or turkey and a green salad with olives, pine nuts, walnuts, grated carrots, tomatoes
Dinner	Any meat or fish with allowed vegetables from FODMAP diet
Thursday	Lactose free yoghurt with fruit from FODMAP list and nuts (almonds, pecans, brazils, hazelnuts, walnuts, cashews)
Lunch	Chicken or turkey broth and allowed FODMAP vegetables
Dinner	Any meat or fish/shellfish with allowed FODMAP vegetables
Friday	Egg and banana pancake
Lunch	Tuna or hard cheese with a mixed salad using FODMAP salad vegetables
Dinner	Salmon and avocado (if tolerated), celery, spinach, tomatoes
Saturday	Bacon, eggs and grilled tomato
Lunch	Lactose free yoghurt with allowed FODMAP fruits
Dinner	Courgetti or carrot 'spaghetti' with grated parmesan cheese, olives, pine nuts, olive oil

Sunday	Lactose free yoghurt with nuts (almonds, pecans, brazils, hazelnuts, walnuts, cashews, chestnuts)
Lunch	Roast Sunday dinner (no Yorkshire pudding, avoid gravy mix), FODMAP allowed vegetables
Dinner	Chicken or turkey broth, only add allowed vegetables from FODMAP diet

Snacking between meals is best avoided, but if a snack is eaten, opt for a low carbohydrate or protein food such as a piece of cooked fish or meat, or nuts.

Therapeutic diet for acne

Monday	Cantaloupe melon and spinach smoothie made with water
Mid-morning	Olives and nuts
Lunch	Tomato soup and oatcakes
Dinner	Baked salmon steak with asparagus, carrots and sweet potato

Tuesday	Mixed fruit salad with berries, mango, apricots, peach and red grapes sprinkled with wheat germ and mixed seeds
Mid-morning	Soy or coconut yoghurt
Lunch	Corn tortilla wrap with bean sprouts, cucumber, radish, onion, watercress and avocado
Dinner	Brown rice vegetable risotto including garlic, onion, corn, peas and peppers

Wednesday	Banana and egg pancakes
Mid-morning	Nut/seed bar
Lunch	Large green salad with mozzarella, vine tomatoes, avocado, rocket, onion, garlic, olives & pine seeds
Dinner	Savoy cabbage/red onion stir fry with tofu, baby corn, mange tout, sesame seeds and pine nuts

Thursday	Soy or coconut yoghurt with added seeds, nectarines, plums
Mid-morning	Oatcakes with raw carrot crudités and hummus
Lunch	Lentil soup
Dinner	Seared tuna with garlic-roasted squash, carrot and broccoli

Friday	Poached egg served on a bed of spinach or seeded bread
Mid-morning	Tomatoes, raw peppers and carrot crudités with hummus
Lunch	Jacket potato with tuna or hummus and a mixed salad
Dinner	Superfood curry with brown rice

Saturday	Granola mixed with cashew nuts and seeds
Snacks	Olives, almonds and Brazil nuts
Lunch	Chick pea and brown rice salad with raisins, pine nuts and mixed salad vegetables
Dinner	Steamed fish or steak with broccoli, garlic-roasted squash and sweet potato

Sunday	Fruit salad with peaches, cantaloupe melon and berries
Mid-morning	Soya yoghurt
Lunch	Roast Sunday dinner
Dinner	Watercress/lentil/pea or broccoli soup

Therapeutic diet for inflammatory skin conditions (eczema and psoriasis)

Monday	Porridge with mixed seeds and raspberries
Mid-morning	Celery, apple, carrot and radish sticks
Lunch	Peppered mackerel with a green leafy salad, beetroot, tomatoes, red onion and grated carrot and avocado
Dinner	Spicy bean chili with brown rice

Tuesday	Fruit salad with mixed berries, mango, apricots, peach, kiwi and red grapes with soy or live yoghurt and mixed seeds
Mid-morning	Celery, carrot and pepper crudités with cherry tomatoes
Lunch	Mixed bean salad with avocado, tomatoes, onions, cucumber, radish and walnuts
Dinner	Tuna or salmon steak with a large salad or with vegetables

Wednesday	Granola (toasted oats and seeds) with cherries and apricots
Mid-morning	A handful of nuts or olives
Lunch	Sardines on whole meal toast with a dark green leafy salad and beetroot
Dinner	Savoy cabbage/red onion stir fry with baby corn, tofu, mange tout, sesame and fenugreek seeds or pine nuts

Thursday	Poached egg with asparagus OR scrambled egg with smoked salmon/spinach
Mid-morning	Handful of nuts or olives
Lunch	Lentil soup and oatcakes
Dinner	Salmon and sweet potato risotto with rocket or spinach

Friday	Porridge with flaked almonds, pumpkin seeds, cherries /berries
Mid-morning	Tomatoes, raw peppers and carrot crudités with hummus
Lunch	Mackerel pate on oatcakes/corn cakes with raw vegetables
Dinner	Tuna steak or sea bass with olive oil roasted squash, sweet potato and carrots, served with broccoli

Saturday	Poached egg on a bed of spinach
Snacks	A handful of cherries or nuts
Lunch	Lentil and vegetable soup and oatcakes
Dinner	Baked fish/organic meat with roast vegetables and cabbage
Sunday	Banana and egg pancakes
Mid-morning	Handful of nuts or olives
Lunch	Roast dinner – use gluten free gravy
Tea	Avocado and salmon with baby potatoes, green leaves, tomatoes, cucumber, celery and radish

... and drink milk-free Oolong tea or green tea.

Appendix B

Recipes

Fruit and vegetable smoothies

For a thicker consistency, add a spoonful of live yoghurt, some ground nuts or half an avocado, or half a banana.

Serves 1

Ingredients

1 handful of spinach
1 handful of EITHER any type of berry, melon or half an orange

Method

1 Mix with a little water and blend the ingredients together in a blender and serve.

Banana and egg pancake

Serves 2

Ingredients

1 banana
2 eggs
Olive or coconut oil

Method

1 Blend the eggs and banana together to make a batter, meanwhile, heat the oil.
2 Add the batter to the hot oil in small pancake sizes.
3 Cook on each side and serve with coconut or live yoghurt, fresh fruit and nuts.

Savoury soufflé

Serves 2

Ingredients

1 onion
2 cloves garlic
2 handfuls of spinach
1 packet of feta cheese — *try half a block, rather strong flavour*
1 egg
Fresh tomatoes

Method

1 Brown an onion and garlic and then wilt in a few handfuls of spinach.
2 Mix this into a bowl with a beaten egg and a pack of feta cheese (or other cheese will do) and some tomatoes (you could add any vegetables).
3 Put into oiled ramekins and bake for 40 minutes at 200°C.

Banana, walnut and cinnamon quinoa

Serves 2

Ingredients

1 very ripe mashed banana
¼ cup uncooked quinoa
¼ cup of milk, any type
2 tablespoons walnuts (or pecans)
¼ teaspoon of cinnamon

Method

1 Cook the quinoa as per pack instructions. Once cooked, stir in all the other ingredients, empty into a bowl and eat whilst warm.
2 You can add the nuts on top if you prefer that to including them in the mix.

Kedgeree

Serves 2

Ingredients

100g brown rice
2 haddock/mackerel fillets
2 organic eggs
1 teaspoon turmeric

Method

1 Cook the rice as usual.
2 Meanwhile poach the fish in water or skimmed milk.
3 Mix the cooked brown rice with the fish and 1 teaspoon of turmeric.
4 Chop the boiled egg on top and add some fresh coriander or dill.

Summer Mediterranean-style sandwich

Serves 2 – 4 depending on the size of the loaf

Ingredients

One loaf of olive, ciabbata or vine tomato bread or individual rolls
One avocado
One packet of low-fat mozzarella cheese
A handful of vine tomatoes
One bag of rocket leaves

Method

1 Halve a loaf of olive or vine tomato bread lengthways
2 Sprinkle with olive oil
3 Mash up a ripe avocado and spread it on the bread.
4 Layer low-fat mozzarella cheese, vine or sun dried tomatoes and rocket leaves on the bottom part of the loaf.
5 Put the top half of the loaf back on and press down.
6 Wrap in greaseproof paper and ideally place something heavy, such as a plate, on top of the sandwich for a few hours to let the flavours infuse and stick the sandwich together.
7 Cut into sandwich chunks and eat.

Tomato soup

Serves 2

Ingredients

1 tablespoon olive oil
1 onion, grated
1 red chili, de-seeded and chopped
2 garlic cloves, crushed
Half a pint of vegetable stock
2 tablespoons chopped parsley, coriander or basil
8 medium tomatoes, chopped

Method

1 Heat the oil and soften the onion
2 Add the chili and garlic and heat for another minute.
3 Add the chopped tomatoes and cook for 10 minutes.
4 Add the stock, bring to the boil and then simmer for 20 minutes (alternatively, this can be cooked in a slow cooker on low for 5 – 6 hours.
5 Puree the soup in a blender and serve, adding the freshly chopped parsley or basil.
6 Any other vegetable can be used in addition to, or instead of the tomatoes. Cooked lentils or beans can be added at the same time as the vegetables, but adding these as well will increase the number of portions.

Salmon and sweet potato risotto

Serves 2

Ingredients

2 salmon steaks
2 cloves garlic, finely diced
One bag or 4 large handfuls of rocket
2 medium-sized sweet potatoes, roasted
1 onion, sliced
150g organic brown rice or risotto
One bag or 4 large handfuls of rocket
Olive oil

Method

1 Bake the salmon steak and roast the sweet potato in olive oil. Meanwhile, cook the risotto as follows: sauté some garlic and onion in a pan with a little olive oil.
2 Add the rice, stirring to coat it with the oil/onion/garlic mixture, then add water and allow to simmer, gradually adding water as required until the rice is cooked. If you have parboiled the sweet potato before roasting, use this water.
3 Once the rice is cooked add the roasted vegetables, rocket and baked salmon to the risotto and serve.

Spring savoy cabbage stir fry

Serves 2

Ingredients

1 onion
2 garlic cloves
1 Savoy cabbage
A handful of mushrooms
A handful of frozen peas
A handful of sweet corn
A handful of mange tout
A handful of peppers
1 portion of tofu, chicken or turkey
½ tin of baked beans or tinned tomatoes

Method

1 Heat a little olive oil in a pan.
2 Add the chopped onion and the cloves of sliced garlic.
3 Any herbs or spices can also be added at this time (such as chopped chilli, turmeric, oregano or ginger).
4 Cut the Savoy cabbage into thin strips and add this to the pan.
5 Once the onion and cabbage are slightly browned, add the other vegetables, mushrooms, frozen peas, sweet corn or baby corn, mange tout and strips of fresh or frozen peppers.
6 Add a portion of tofu, chicken or turkey, and half a tin of baked beans or tinned tomatoes can be used to create a sauce – just add to the mix and stir until heated through.

Chilli bean casserole

Serves 4

Ingredients

A selection of beans/lentils, soaked – choose from any type of beans and lentils, and combine a selection to make up 200g-250g dry weight
1 onion, chopped
2 cloves of garlic, chopped
1-2 chillies, chopped
A handful of mushrooms
2 carrots, diced
A handful of frozen peas and sweet corn
A handful of fresh/frozen peppers
1 tin of tomatoes
A cupful of fresh tomatoes
60g organic brown rice per person

Method

1 Soak a selection of beans overnight.
2 While boiling the beans for the designated amount of time, brown the onion and garlic in a little olive oil then add the fresh chillies.
3 Add the mushrooms, carrots and other vegetables to the dish with the tinned tomatoes.
4 Simmer for one hour, adding the beans halfway through.
5 If pre-cooked beans or lentils are being used, add them to the chilli to provide the recommended cooking time. Fresh tomatoes may also be added later on.
6 Serve with brown rice.

Superfood curry

Serves 2

Ingredients

1 tsp olive oil
2 cloves garlic
1 onion
Handful of fresh coriander
2 tsp turmeric

2 red chillies, chopped — *hot, try one !*
1 carrots
1 large sweet potato
3 large fresh tomatoes
1 vegetable stock cube made into 300ml
1 small tin of chickpeas
1 head of broccoli
1 small pot fat-free Greek yoghurt

Method

1 Heat the oil, cooking the garlic and onion until soft.

2 Add a tsp of finely chopped coriander, the turmeric and chillies.

3 Stir and cook for two minutes.

4 Add carrots, sweet potato and tomatoes.

5 Add the liquid stock and chickpeas, bring to the boil and then simmer for approximately 20 minutes.

6 Meanwhile, blanch the broccoli and add once the curry is cooked. Remove from the heat; allow to cool slightly before adding the yoghurt.

7 Sprinkle a generous helping of fresh coriander on top and serve on its own or with brown rice (60g per person, uncooked weight).

Stuffed vegetables

Serves 2

Ingredients

2 potatoes
1 tsp of olive oil
2 cloves of garlic, chopped
1 handful each of mushrooms, fresh or frozen sweetcorn and peas
1 onion, chopped
100g fresh spinach
2 large peppers, raw, with tops cut off
1 dessertspoon of mixed seeds – pumpkin, sunflower and sesame seeds
Green salad

Method

1 Bake the potatoes until cooked.
2 Meanwhile, heat a little oil and lightly stir fry the garlic, mushroom and onion.
3 Add the seeds, peas and sweet corn and heat through, adding the spinach.
4 Stir until wilted and remove from the heat.
5 Cut off the top of the potatoes and scoop out the mash into the stir fry and mix.
6 Once thoroughly mixed, stuff the peppers and potatoes with the mixture of stir-fried onions, garlic, mushrooms, peas, spinach, sweet corn, and mixed seeds and bake for 35 minutes at to 180°C/356°F/Gas Mark 4.
7 Serve with a large green salad.

Seared tuna steak with stir fry vegetables

Try swapping tuna steak for swordfish or marlin steaks in this recipe.

Serves 2

Ingredients

1 handful of mushrooms
2 cloves of garlic
1 onion
1 tsp olive oil
1 fresh pepper
1 cupful of mixed sweet corn and peas
1 tsp sesame seeds
2 tuna steaks

Method

1 Chop the mushrooms, garlic and onions and add to a tsp of heated olive oil in a pan.
2 Once browned, add the chopped peppers, sweet corn and peas, and cook through.
3 Add the seeds and heat for a further few minutes until just browned.
4 Meanwhile, sear the tuna steak in a non-stick pan. You could rub chopped chilli and garlic onto the fish beforehand if you wish.
5 Serve the vegetables and tuna together.

Help List

Organisations

Arthritis Care

Arthritis Care, 18 Stephenson Way, London NW1 2HD
Tel: 020 7380 6500
Info@arthritiscare.org.uk
www.arthritiscare.org.uk
Arthritis Care is the UK's largest charity organisation for people with arthritis. The website provides information on arthritis, events and news.

British Heart Foundation

British Heart Foundation, Greater London House, 180 Hampstead Road, London NW1 7AW
Tel: 020 7554 0000
Fax: 020 7554 0100
www.bhf.org.uk

British Association for Applied Nutrition and Nutritional Therapy (BANT)

British Association for Applied Nutrition and Nutritional Therapy
27 Old Gloucester Street, London WC1N 3XX
Telephone: 08706 061284
www.bant.org.uk
BANT is a professional body for nutritional therapists and those working in the field of nutritional science. A list of registered practitioners can be found on the BANT website.

Complementary and Natural Healthcare Council (CNHC)

The CNHC is the UK voluntary regulator for nutritional therapists.
https://www.cnhc.org.uk

British Heart Foundation

British Heart Foundation, Greater London House, 180 Hampstead Road, London NW1 7AW
Tel: 020 7554 0000
Fax: 020 7554 0100
Heart HelpLine: 0300 330 3311 (open Monday to Friday 9am-6pm)
internet@bhf.org.uk
www.bhf.org.uk

British Nutrition Foundation

High Holborn House, 52-54 High Holborn. London. WC1V 6RQ
Tel: 0207 4046504
postbox@nutrition.org.uk This e-mail address is being protected from spambots. You need JavaScript enabled to view it
www.nutrition.org.uk
The British Nutrition Foundation is a credible source of nutrition information. It provides reliable information on food, nutrition and healthy eating, as well as topical news items and scientific research.

Diabetes UK Central Office

Diabetes UK, Macleod House, 10 Parkway, London NW1 7AA
Tel: 020 7424 1000
Fax: 020 7424 1001
Email info@diabetes.org.uk
https://www.diabetes.org.uk

Dr. Axe – Nightshade foods

Find further information and a list of Nightshade foods here:
https://draxe.com/nightshade-vegetables/

Eatwell

https://www.nhs.uk/live-well/eat-well/the-eatwell-guide/
The NHS eatwell website provides a wealth of trustworthy, practical information about food and healthy eating such as tips on what to eat for a healthy heart, how to help prevent osteoporosis, and which foods may boost mental function.

Food and Behaviour Research

Food and Behaviour Research (FAB Research), established in 2003, is a charitable organisation dedicated both to advancing scientific research into the links between nutrition and human behaviour and to making the findings from such research available to the widest possible audience. A plethora of information and research articles can be found here, specially on the effects of diet on mental health.
FAB Research, 163 Woodford Road, Woodford, Cheshire SK71QD
Telephone: 07434 185 525
admin@fabresearch.org
https://www.fabresearch.org/viewItem.php

National Osteoporosis Society

National Osteoporosis Society, Camerton, Bath BA2 0PJ

Tel: 01761 471771 / 0845 130 3076

Helpline: 0845 450 0230

www.nos.org.uk

Email: info@nos.org.uk

NHS

Visit this NHS website for information on various health conditions.

https://www.nhs.uk/conditions/

The Cholesterol Truth

A website providing information on alternatives to cholesterol lowering medication.

http://www.thecholesteroltruth.com

UK Gout Society Secretariat

PO Box 90, Hindhead, GU27 9FW

Email: info@ukgoutsociety.org

Book list

Acid and Alkaline
By Herman Aihara. George Ohsawa Macrobiotic Foundation 1986.

Foods that Harm, Foods that Heal
By Readers Digest, Readers Digest Assoc., 2004.
A useful guide to foods to eat and foods to avoid for a wide range of conditions.

Encyclopedia of Natural Medicine
By Michael Murray and Joseph Pizzorno, Three Rivers Press, 1998.

GI How to succeed using a Glycaemic Index diet
By Harper Collins, HarperCollins Publishers, Glasgow, 2005.
A comprehensive guide to the glycaemic index of foods.

Teach Yourself Lose Weight, Gain Energy, Get Healthy
By Sara Kirkham, Hodder, 2010
A topical guide to detoxing, eating a superfood diet and re-charging your energy levels with therapeutic and exclusion diets to follow.

The Mediterranean Diet
By Marissa Cloutier and Eve Adamson, HarperCollins, 2004.

The Optimum Nutrition Bible
By Patrick Holford. Piatkus,1997.

The PK Cookbook
Dr. Sarah Myhill and Craig Robinson. Hammersmith Health Books, London.
For an overview of ketosis, recipes and a very simplified, easy way of eating on a ketogenic diet.

Vitamin D: Physiology, Molecular Biology, and Clinical Applications
By Michael F. Holick, Humana Press, 1998.
For in depth information on vitamin D and its effects upon osteoporosis and skin diseases.

Weight Loss – The Essential Guide
By Sara Kirkham, Need2Know, 2019
The ultimate guide to helping you lose weight and improve your health with a superfood diet.

What colour is your diet
By David Heber, HarperCollins, 2001.
An interesting book packed with information on the phytonutrients in food.

Journal articles

Heart disease

Alphonse PA, Ramprasath V, Jones PJ. 'Effect of dietary cholesterol and plant sterol consumption on plasma lipid responsiveness and cholesterol trafficking in healthy individuals'. *British Journal of Nutrition*, 2017, Volume 117(1):56-66.

Batuca JR, Amaral MC, Favas C, Paula FS, Ames PRJ, Papoila AL, Delgado Alves J. 'Extended-release niacin increases anti-apolipoprotein A-I antibodies that block the antioxidant effect of high-density lipoprotein-cholesterol: the EXPLORE clinical trial'. *British Journal of Clinical Pharmacology*, 2017, Volume 83(5):1002-1010.

Buckley D, Muench J, Hamilton A. How effective are dietary interventions in lowering lipids in adults with dyslipidemia? *The Journal of Family Practice*, 2007, Volume 56, Issue 1: 46-48.

Buscemi S, Verga S, Batsis JA, Donatelli M, Tranchina MR, Belmonte S, Mattina A, Re A, Cerasola G. 'Acute effects of coffee on endothelial function in healthy subjects'. *European Journal of Clinical Nutrition,* 2010, Volume 64, Issue 5: 483-9.

Cavagnaro PF, Camargo A, Galmarini CR, Simon PW. 'Effect of cooking on garlic (Allium sativum L.) antiplatelet activity and thiosulfinates content'. *Journal of Agricultural and Food Chemistry,* 2007, Volume 55, Issue 4: 1280-8.

Chei CL, Loh JK, Soh A, Yuan JM, Koh WP. 'Coffee, tea, caffeine, and risk of hypertension: The Singapore Chinese Health Study'. *European Journal of Nutrition*, 2017. Volume 56(1): 1-12.

Dehghan *et al*, 'Associations of fats and carbohydrate intake with cardiovascular disease and mortality in 18 countries from five continents (PURE): a prospective cohort study'. *The Lancet*, 2017, Volume 390 (10107):2050-2062.

Duggal JK, Singh M, Attri N, Singh PP, Ahmed N, Pahwa S, Molnar J, Singh S, Khosla S, Arora R. 'Effect of niacin therapy on cardiovascular outcomes in patients with coronary artery disease'. *Journal of Cardiovascular Pharmacology and Therapeutics,* 2010, Volume 15, Issue 2: 158-66.

Eyres L, Eyres MF, Chisholm A and Brown RC. Coconut oil consumption and cardiovascular risk factors in humans. *Nutrition Reviews*, 2016, Volume 74(4):267-80. doi: 10.1093/nutrit/nuw002.

Hertog MG, Feskens EJ, Hollman PC, Katan MB, Kromhout D. 'Dietary antioxidant flavonoids and risk of coronary heart disease: the Zutphen Elderly Study'. *Lancet*, 1993, Volume 342, Issue 8878: 1007-11.

Jialal I , Grundy SM. 'Effect of dietary supplementation with alpha-tocopherol on the oxidative modification of low density lipoprotein'. Journal of Lipid Research,1992, Volume 33(6):899-906.

Jenkins DJ, Kendall CW, Marchie A, Faulkner DA, Wong JM, de Souza R, Emam A, Parker TL, Vidgen E, Trautwein EA, Lapsley KG, Josse RG, Leiter LA, Singer W, Connelly PW. 'Direct comparison of a dietary portfolio of cholesterol-lowering foods with a statin in hypercholesterolemic participants'. *The American Journal of Clinical Nutrition*, 2005, Volume 81, Issue 2: 380-387.

Khaw KT, Sharp SJ, Finikarides L, Afzal I, Lentjes M, Luben R and Forouhi NG. Randomised trial of coconut oil, olive oil or butter on blood lipids and other cardiovascular risk factors in healthy men and women. *BMJ Open*, 2018, Volume 6;8(3):e020167.

Key TJ, Fraser GE, Thorogood M, Appleby PN, Beral V, Reeves G, Burr ML, Chang-Claude J, Frentzel-Beyme R, Kuzma JW, Mann J, McPherson K. 'Mortality in vegetarians and non-vegetarians: a collaborative analysis of 8300 deaths among 76,000 men and women in five prospective studies'. *Public Health Nutrition*, 1998, Volume 1, Issue 1: 33-41.

Lekakis J, Rallidis LS, Andreadou I, Vamvakou G, Kazantzoglou G, Magiatis P, Skaltsounis AL and Kremastinos DT. 'Polyphenolic compounds from red grapes acutely improve endothelial function in patients with coronary heart disease'. *European Journal of Cardiovascular Prevention and Rehabilitation*, 2005, Volume 12, Issue 6: 596-600.

Manolopoulos KN, Karpe F, Frayn KN. 'Gluteofemoral body fat as a determinant of metabolic health'. *International Journal of Obesity,* 2010, Volume 34(6):949-59.

Mensink RP and Katan MB. 'Effect of dietary fatty acids on serum lipids and lipoproteins. A meta-analysis of 27 trials'. *Arteriosclerosis and Thrombosis*, 1992, Volume 12, Issue 8: 911-9.

Mineharu Y, Koizumi A, Wada Y, Iso H, Watanabe Y, Date C, Yamamoto A, Kikuchi S, Inaba Y, Toyoshima H, Kondo T, Tamakoshi A. 'Coffee, green tea, black tea and oolong tea consumption and risk of mortality from cardiovascular disease in Japanese men and women'. *Journal of Epidemiology and Community Health*, 2011, Volume 65(3):230-40.

Moore TJ, Alsabeeh N, Apovian CM, Murphy MC, Coffman GA, Cullum-Dugan D, Jenkins M, Cabral H. 'Weight, blood pressure, and dietary benefits after 12 months of a Web-based Nutrition Education Program (DASH for health): longitudinal observational study'. *Journal of Medical Internet Research,* 2008, Volume 10, Issue 4: 52.

Moreyra AE, Wilson AC, Koraym A. 'Effect of combining psyllium fiber with simvastatin in lowering cholesterol'. *Archives of Internal Medicine,* 2005, Volume 165, Issue 10 :1161-6.

Mortensen SA, Rosenfeldt F, Kumar A, Dolliner P, Filipiak KJ, Pella D6, Alehagen U, Steurer G, Littarru GP; Q-SYMBIO Study Investigators. 'The effect of coenzyme Q10 on morbidity and mortality in chronic heart failure: results from Q-SYMBIO: a randomized double-blind trial'. *JACC. Heart Failure*, 2014 Volume 2(6):641-9.

Mottillo S, Filion KB, Genest J, Joseph L, Pilote L, Poirier P, Rinfret S, Schiffrin EL, Eisenberg MJ. The Metabolic Syndrome and Cardiovascular Risk. *The Journal of the American College of Cardiology*, 2010, Volume 56, Issue 14: 1113 – 1132.

Naumann E, van Rees AB, Onning G, Oste R, Wydra M, Mensink RP. 'Beta-glucan incorporated into a fruit drink effectively lowers serum LDL-cholesterol concentrations'. *American Journal of Clinical Nutrition*, 2006, Volume 83, Issue 3: 601-5.

Ostlund RE Jr, Racette SB, Okeke A, Stenson WF. Phytosterols that are naturally present in commercial corn oil significantly reduce cholesterol absorption in humans'. *The American Journal of Clinical Nutrition*, 2002, Volume 75(6):1000-4.

Othman RA, Moghadasian MH, Jones PJ. 'Cholesterol-lowering effects of oat []-glucan'. *Nutrition Reviews*, 2011, Volume 69(6):299-309. doi: 10.1111/j.1753-4887.2011.00401.x.

Ravid Z, Bendayan M, Delvin E, Sane AT, Elchebly M, Lafond J, Lambert M, Mailhot MG, Levy E 'Modulation of intestinal cholesterol absorption by high glucose levels: impact on cholesterol transporters, regulatory enzymes, and transcription factors'. *American Journal of Physiology – Gastrointestinal and Liver Physiology*, 2008, Volume 295, Issue 5: G873-G885.

Remig V, Franklin B, Margolis S, Kostas G, Nece T and Street JC. 'Trans fats in America: a review of their use, consumption, health implications, and regulation'. *Journal of the American Dietetic Association*, 2010, Volume 110, Issue 4:585-92.

Siavash M and Amini M. 'Vitamin C may have similar beneficial effects to Gemfibrozil on serum high-density lipoprotein-cholesterol in type 2 diabetic patients'. *Journal of Research in Pharmacy Practice*. 2014, Volume 3(3):77-82.

Siri-Tarino PW, Sun Q, Hu FB, Krauss RM. 'Meta-analysis of prospective cohort studies evaluating the association of saturated fat with cardiovascular disease'. *The American Journal of Clinical Nutrition*, 2010, Volume 91, Issue 3: 535-46.

Sobenin IA, Andrianova IV, Fomchenkov IV, Gorchakova TV, Orekhov AN. 'Time-released garlic powder tablets lower systolic and diastolic blood pressure in men with mild and moderate arterial hypertension'. *Hypertension Research*. 2009, Volume 32, Issue 6: 433-7.

Sood N, Baker WL, Coleman CI. 'Effect of glucomannan on plasma lipid and glucose concentrations, body weight, and blood pressure: systematic review and meta-analysis'. *The American Journal of Clinical Nutrition,* 2008, Volume 88, Issue 4: 1167-75.

Tang F, Lu M, Zhang S, Mei M, Wang T, Liu P, Wang H. 'Vitamin E conditionally inhibits atherosclerosis in ApoE knockout mice by anti-oxidation and regulation of vasculature gene expressions'. *Lipids.* 2014, Volume 49(12):1215-23.

Tverdal A, Magnus P, Selmer R, Thelle D. Consumption of alcohol and cardiovascular disease mortality: a 16 year follow-up of 115,592 Norwegian men and women aged 40-44 years. *European Journal of Epidemiology,* 2017, Volume 32(9):775-783.

Yuen KH, Wong JW, Lim AB, Ng BH, Choy WP. 'Effect of Mixed-Tocotrienols in Hypercholesterolemic Subjects'. *Functional Foods in Health and Disease*, 2011, Volume 3:106-117.

Yzebe D, and Lievre M. 'Fish oils in the care of coronary heart disease patients: a meta-analysis of randomized controlled trials'. Fundamental and Clinical *Pharmacology,* 2004, Volume 18, Issue 5: 581-92.

Zeng T, Guo FF, Zhang CL, Song FY, Zhao XL, Xie KQ. 'A meta-analysis of randomized, double-blind, placebo-controlled trials for the effects of garlic on serum lipid profiles'. *Journal of the Science of Food and Agriculture, 2012.*

Arthritis, osteoporosis and gout

Abdel-Rahman MS, Alkady EA, Ahmed S. 'Menaquinone-7 as a novel pharmacological therapy in the treatment of rheumatoid arthritis: A clinical study'. *European Journal of Pharmacology,* 2015, Volume 15;761:273-8.

Abdulrazaq M, Innes JK, Calder PC. 'Effect of ￿-3 polyunsaturated fatty acids on arthritic pain: A systematic review'. *Nutrition*, 2017, Volume 39-40:57-66.

Adam O, Beringer C, Kless T, Lemmen C, Adam A, Wiseman M, Adam P, Klimmek R. and Forth W. 'Anti-inflammatory effects of a low arachidonic acid diet and fish oil in patients with rheumatoid arthritis'. *Rheumatology International,* 2003, Volume 23, Issue 1: 27-36.

Akbar U, Yang M, Kurian D, Mohan C. 'Omega-3 Fatty Acids in Rheumatic Diseases: A Critical Review'. *Journal of Clinical Rheumatology*, 2017, Volume 23(6):330-339.

Ameye LG and Chee WS 'Osteoarthritis and nutrition. From nutraceuticals to functional foods: a systematic review of the scientific evidence'. *Arthritis research and Therapy*, 2008, Volume 8, Issue 4: 1-22.

Aryaeian N, Djalali M, Shahram F, Jazayeri Sh, Chamari M, Nazari S. 'Beta-Carotene, Vitamin E, MDA, Glutathione Reductase and Arylesterase Activity Levels in Patients with Active Rheumatoid Arthritis'. *Iranian Journal of Public Health*, 2011, Volume 40(2):102-9.

Berg KM, Kunins HV, Jackson JL, Nahvi S, Chaudhry A, Harris KA, Malik R. and Arnsten JH. 'Association Between Alcohol Consumption and Both Osteoporotic Fracture and Bone Density'. *The American Journal of Medicine*, 2008, Volume 121, Issue 5: 406-418.

Blau LW. 'Cherry diet control for gout and arthritis'.*Texas Reports on Biology and Medicine*, 1950, Volume 8(3):309-11.

Bolland MJ, Leung W, Tai V, Bastin S, Gamble GD, Grey A, Reid IR. 'Calcium intake and risk of fracture: systematic review'. *British Medical Journal*, 2015, Volume 29;351:h4580.

Buchanan HM, Preston SJ, Brooks PM and Buchanan WW. 'Is diet important in rheumatoid arthritis?' *British Journal of Rheumatology*, 1991, Volume 30, Issue 2: 125-34.

Cameron M, Gagnier JJ, Chrubasik S, 'Herbal therapy for treating rheumatoid arthritis'. *The Cochrane Database of Systematic Reviews*, 2011, Volume 16;(2):CD002948.

Choi HK, Gao X, Curhan G. 'Vitamin C Intake and the Risk of Gout in Men – A Prospective Study'. *Archives of Internal Medicine*, 2009, Volume 9; 169(5): 502–507.

Cohen A, Goldman J. 'Bromelains therapy in rheumatoid arthritis', *Pennsylvania Medical Journal,* 1964, Volume 67:27–30.

Daily JW, Yang M, Park S. 'Efficacy of Turmeric Extracts and Curcumin for Alleviating the Symptoms of Joint Arthritis: A Systematic Review and Meta-Analysis of Randomized Clinical Trials'. *Journal of Medicinal Food*, 2016, Volume 1; 19(8): 717–729.

Dalbeth N, Palmano K. 'Effects of dairy intake on hyperuricemia and gout'. *Current Rheumatology Reports*, 2011, Volume 13(2):132-7.

Ebina K, Shi K, Hirao M, Kaneshiro S, Morimoto T, Koizumi K, Yoshikawa H, Hashimoto J. 'Vitamin K2 administration is associated with decreased disease activity in patients with rheumatoid arthritis'. *Modern Rheumatology*, 2013, Volume 23(5):1001-7.

Jacob R.A., Spinozzi G.M., Simon V.A., Kelley D.S., Prior R.L., Hess-Pierce B., Kader A.A. 'Consumption of cherries lowers plasma urate in healthy women'. *Journal of Nutrition*, 2003, Volume 133:1826–1829.

Johnson SA, Feresin RG, Soung do Y, Elam ML, Arjmandi BH. 'Vitamin E suppresses ex vivo osteoclastogenesis in ovariectomized rats'. *Food and Function,* 2016, Volume 7(3):1628-33.

Juraschek SP, Edgar R. Miller ER, Gelber AC 'Effect of Oral Vitamin C Supplementation on Serum Uric Acid: A Meta-analysis of Randomized Controlled Trials'. *Arthritis Care and Research*, 2011, Volume 63(9): 1295–1306.

Karatay S, Erdem T, Yildirim K, Melikoglu MA, Ugur M, Cakir E, Akcay F, Senel K. 'The effect of individualized diet challenges consisting of allergenic foods on TNF-alpha and IL-1beta levels in patients with rheumatoid arthritis.' *Rheumatology,* 2004, Volume 43, Issue 11: 429-33.

Karatay S, Erdem T, Kiziltunc A, Melikoglu MA, Yildirim K, Cakir E, Ugur M, Aktas A and Senel K. 'General or personal diet: the individualized model for diet challenges in patients with rheumatoid arthritis'. *Rheumatology International*, 2006, Volume 26, Issue 6: 556-60.

Kargutkar S, Brijesh S. 'Anti-rheumatic activity of Ananas comosus fruit peel extract in a complete Freund's adjuvant rat model'. *Pharmaceutical biology*, 2016, Volume 54(11):2616-2622.

Karlson EW, Shadick NA, Cook NR, Buring JE, Lee IM. 'Vitamin E in the primary prevention of rheumatoid arthritis: the Women's Health Study'. *Arthritis and Rheumatism,* 2008, Volume15;59(11):1589-95.

Kasemsuk T, Saengpetch N, Sibmooh N, Unchern S. 'Improved WOMAC score following 16-week treatment with bromelain for knee osteoarthritis'. *Clinical Rheumatology,* 2016, Volume 35(10):2531-40.

Lee YH, Bae SC, 'Vitamin D level in rheumatoid arthritis and its correlation with the disease activity: a meta-analysis'. *Clinical and experimental rheumatology,* 2016. Volume 34(5):827-833.

Merlino LA, Curtis J, Mikuls TR, Cerhan JR, Criswell LA, Saag KG; Iowa Women's Health Study. 'Vitamin D intake is inversely associated with rheumatoid arthritis: results from the Iowa Women's Health Study'. *Arthritis and Rheumatism*, 2004, Volume 50, Issue 1: 72-7.

Rønn SH, Harsløf T, Pedersen SB, Langdahl BL 'Vitamin K2 (menaquinone-7) prevents age-related deterioration of trabecular bone microarchitecture at the tibia in postmenopausal women'. *European Journal of Endocrinology*, 2016, Volume 175(6):541-549.

Scientific Advisory Committee on Nutrition (2016) *Vitamin D and Health*. Available at: < https://assets.publishing.service.gov.uk/government/uploads/system/uploads/attachment_data/file/537616/SACN_Vitamin_D_and_Health_report.pdf>.

Sawitzke AD, Shi H, Finco MF, Dunlop DD, Bingham CO 3rd, Harris CL, Singer NG, Bradley JD, Silver D, Jackson CG, Lane NE, Oddis CV, Wolfe F, Lisse J, Furst DE, Reda DJ, Moskowitz RW, Williams HJ, Clegg DO. 'The effect of glucosamine and/or chondroitin sulfate on the progression of knee osteoarthritis: a report from the glucosamine/chondroitin arthritis intervention trial'. *Journal of Arthritis and Rheumatism*, 2008, Volume 58, Issue 10: 3183-91.

Smedslund G, Byfuglien MG, Olsen SU, Hagen KB. Effectiveness and safety of dietary interventions for rheumatoid arthritis: a systematic review of randomized controlled trials. *Journal of the American Dietetic Association*, 2010, Volume 110(5):727-35.

Torralba KD, De Jesus E, Rachabattula S. 'The interplay between diet, urate transporters and the risk for gout and hyperuricemia: current and future directions'. *International Journal of Rheumatic Diseases*, 2012, Volume 15(6):499-506.

Zhang Z, Leong DL, Xu, L, Hc Z, Wang A, Navati M, Kirn SJ, Hirsh DM, Hardin JA, Cobelli NJ, Friedman JM, Sun HB. 'Curcumin slows osteoarthritis progression and relieves osteoarthritis-associated pain symptoms in a post-traumatic osteoarthritis mouse model'. *Arthritis Research and Therapy*, 2016, Volume18: 128.

Zhang Y, Neogi T, Chen C, Chaisson C, Hunter DJ, Choi HK. Cherry consumption and decreased risk of recurrent gout attacks. *Arthritis and Rheumatism*, 2012, Volume 64(12):4004-11.

Diabetes and blood glucose control

Abutair AS, Naser IA, Hamed AT, 'Soluble fibers from psyllium improve glycemic response and body weight among diabetes type 2 patients (randomized control trial)'. *Nutrition Journal*, 2016, Volume 15: 86.

Ang M, Müller AS, Wagenlehner F, Pilatz A, Linn T. Combining protein and carbohydrate increases postprandial insulin levels but does not improve glucose response in patients with type 2 diabetes'. *Metabolism*, 2012, Volume 61(12):1696-702.

Bhupathiraju SN, Pan A, Malik VS, Manson JE, Willett WC, van Dam RM, Hu FB. 'Caffeinated and caffeine-free beverages and risk of type 2 diabetes'. *American Journal of Clinical Nutrition*, 2013, Volume 97(1):155-66.

Cullmann M, Hilding A, Östenson CG. 'Alcohol consumption and risk of pre-diabetes and type 2 diabetes development in a Swedish population'. Diabet Med. *Diabetic medicine*, 2012, Volume 29(4):441-52.

Dixon JB, O'Brien PE, Playfair J *et al* 'Adjustable gastric banding and conventional therapy for type 2 diabetes: a randomized controlled trial'. *JAMA,* 2008, Volume 299:316–323.

Gaddam A, Galla C, Thummisetti S, Marikanty RK, Palanisamy UD, Rao PV, 'Role of Fenugreek in the prevention of type 2 diabetes mellitus in prediabetes'. *Journal of Diabetes and Metabolic Disorders*, 2015, Volume 14: 74.

Huang J, Wang X, Zhang Y. 'Specific types of alcoholic beverage consumption and risk of type 2 diabetes: A systematic review and meta-analysis'. *Journal of Diabetes Investigation*, 2017, Volume 8(1):56-68.

Imamura F, O'Connor L, Ye Z, Mursu J, Hayashino Y, Bhupathiraju SN, Forouhi NG. 'Consumption of sugar sweetened beverages, artificially sweetened beverages, and fruit juice and incidence of type 2 diabetes: systematic review, meta-analysis, and estimation of population attributable fraction'. *British Medical Journal*, 2015, Volume 21;351:h3576.

Jamilian M, Zadeh Modarres S, Amiri Siavashani M, Karimi M, Mafi A, Ostadmohammadi V, Asemi Z. 'The Influences of Chromium Supplementation on Glycemic Control, Markers of Cardio-Metabolic Risk, and Oxidative Stress in Infertile Polycystic ovary Syndrome Women Candidate for In vitro Fertilization: a Randomized, Double-Blind, Placebo-Controlled Trial'. *Biological Trace Element Research*, 2018,

Jung CH, Choi KM. 'Impact of High-Carbohydrate Diet on Metabolic Parameters in Patients with Type 2 Diabetes'. *Nutrients*, 2017, Volume 24;9(4). pii: E322.

Kirkham S, Akilen R, Sharma S. and Tsiami A. 'The potential of cinnamon to reduce blood glucose levels in patients with type 2 diabetes and insulin resistance'. *Diabetes, Obesity and Metabolism*, 2009, Volume 11, Issue 12: 1100-1113.

Knott C, Bell S, Britton A. 'Alcohol Consumption and the Risk of Type 2 Diabetes: A Systematic Review and Dose-Response Meta-analysis of More Than 1.9 Million Individuals From 38 Observational Studies'. *Diabetes Care*, 2015, Volume 38(9):1804-12.

Lennerz BS, Barton A, Bernstein RK, Dikeman RD, Diulus C, Hallberg S, Rhodes ET, Ebbeling CB, Westman EC, Yancy WS Jr, Ludwig DS. 'Management of Type 1 Diabetes With a Very Low-Carbohydrate Diet'. *Pediatrics*, 2018, Volume 7, pii: e20173349.

Lim EL, Hollingsworth KG, Aribisala BS, Chen MJ, Mathers JC, Taylor R. 'Reversal of Type 2 Diabetes', 2011, *Diabetologia*, Volume 54:2506–2514.

Linn T, Santosa B, Grönemeyer D, Aygen S, Scholz N, Busch M, Bretzel RG. 'Effect of long-term dietary protein intake on glucose metabolism in humans'. *Diabetologia,* 2000, Volume 43(10):1257-65.

McIlduff CE, Rutkove SB, 'Critical appraisal of the use of alpha lipoic acid (thioctic acid) in the treatment of symptomatic diabetic polyneuropathy'. *Therapeutics and Clinical Risk Management*, 2011, Volume 7: 377–385.

Mitri J and Pittas AG, 'Vitamin D and diabetes', *Endocrinology and Metabolism Clinics of North America*, 2014, Volume 43(1):205-232.

Montonen J, Järvinen R, Heliövaara M, Reunanen A, Aromaa A, Knekt P. 'Food consumption and the incidence of type II diabetes mellitus'. *European Journal of Clinical Nutrition*, 2005, Volume 59, pages 441–448.

Neelakantan N, Narayanan M, de Souza RJ, van Dam RM, 'Effect of fenugreek (*Trigonella foenum-graecum* L.) intake on glycemia: a meta-analysis of clinical trials'. *Nutrition Journal*, 2014, Voume 13: 7.

Patel PS, Forouhi NG, Kuijsten A, *et al*. 'The prospective association between total and type of fish intake and type 2 diabetes in 8 European countries: EPIC-InterAct Study'. *American Journal of Clinical Nutrition*, 2012, Volume 95:1445–1453.

Pories WJ, Caro JF, Flickinger EG, Meelheim HD, Swanson MS 'The control of diabetes mellitus (NIDDM) in the morbidly obese with the Greenville Gastric Bypass', 1987, *Annals of Surgery*, Volume 206:316–323.

Rebelo I, Casal S. 'Coffee: A Dietary Intervention on Type 2 Diabetes?' *Current Medicinal Chemistry*, 2017, Volume 24(4):376-383.

Sluijs I, Beulens JWJ, van der A DL, Spijkerman AMW, Grobbee DE, van der Schouw YT. 'Dietary Intake of Total, Animal, and Vegetable Protein and Risk of Type 2 Diabetes in the European Prospective Investigation into Cancer and Nutrition (EPIC)-NL Study'. *Diabetes Care* 2010, Volume 33(1): 43-48.

Taylor R. 'Banting Memorial lecture 2012: reversing the twin cycles of type 2 diabetes'. *Diabetic Medicine*, 2013, Volume 30(3):267-75.

Tay J, Luscombe-Marsh ND, Thompson CH, Noakes M, Buckley JD, Wittert GA, Yancy WS Jr, Brinkworth GD. 'Comparison of low- and high-carbohydrate diets for type 2 diabetes management: a randomized trial'. *The American Journal of Clinical Nutrition*, 2015, Volume 102(4):780-90.

Tay J, Thompson CH, Luscombe-Marsh ND, Wycherley TP, Noakes M, Buckley JD, Wittert GA, Yancy WS Jr, Brinkworth GD. 'Effects of an energy-restricted low-carbohydrate, high unsaturated fat/low saturated fat diet versus a high-carbohydrate, low-fat diet in type 2 diabetes: A 2-year randomized clinical trial'. *Diabetes, Obesity and Metabolism*, 2018, Volume 20(4):858-871.

van Nielen M, Feskens EJ, Mensink M, Sluijs I, Molina E, Amiano P, Ardanaz E, Balkau B, Beulens JW, Boeing H, Clavel-Chapelon F, Fagherazzi G9, Franks PW, Halkjaer J, Huerta JM, Katzke V, Key TJ, Khaw KT, Krogh V, Kühn T, Menéndez VV, Nilsson P, Overvad K, Palli D, Panico S, Rolandsson O, Romieu I, Sacerdote C, Sánchez MJ, Schulze MB, Spijkerman AM, Tjonneland A, Tumino R, van der A DL, Würtz AM, Zamora-Ros R, Langenberg C, Sharp SJ, Forouhi NG, Riboli E, Wareham NJ; InterAct Consortium. 'Dietary protein intake and incidence of type 2 diabetes in Europe: the EPIC-InterAct Case-Cohort Study'. *Diabetes Care*, 2014, Volume 37(7):1854-62.

Wilson EA, Hadden DR, Merrett JD, Montgomery DA, Weaver JA. 'Dietary management of maturity-onset diabetes'. *British Medical Journal*, 1980, Volume 7;280(6228):1367-9.

Mental function and mood

Almeida OP, Ford AH, Hirani V, Singh V, vanBockxmeer FM, McCaul K, Flicker L. 'B vitamins to enhance treatment response to antidepressants in middle-aged and older adults: results from the B-VITAGE randomised, double-blind, placebo-controlled trial'. *British Journal of Psychiatry*, 2014, Volume 205(6):450-7.

Barnes J, Anderson LA, Phillipson JD. 'St John's wort (Hypericum perforatum L.): a review of its chemistry, pharmacology and clinical properties.' *Journal of Pharmacy and Pharmocology*, 2001, Volume 53(5):583-600.

Beydoun MA, Beydoun HA, Gamaldo AA, Teel A, Zonderman AB, Wang Y, 'Epidemiologic studies of modifiable factors associated with cognition and dementia: systematic review and meta-analysis'. *BMC Public Health.* 2014, Volume 14: 643.

Canevelli M, Adali N, Kelaiditi E, Cantet C, Ousset PJ, Cesari M; ICTUS/DSA Group. 'Effects of Gingko biloba supplementation in Alzheimer's disease patients receiving cholinesterase inhibitors: data from the ICTUS study'. *Phytomedcine,* 2014, Volume 15;21(6):888-92.

Cipriani, A *et al*, 'Comparative efficacy and acceptability of 21 antidepressant drugs for the acute treatment of adults with major depressive disorder: a systematic review and network meta-analysis'. *The Lancet*, 2018, Volume 391 (10128);1357–1366,

Dai Q, Borenstein AR, Wu Y, Jackson JC, Larson EB. 'Fruit and vegetable juices and Alzheimer's disease: the Kame Project'. *American Journal of Medicine*, 2006, Volume 119(9):751-9.

Grosso G, Pajak A, Marventano S, Castellano S, Galvano F, Bucolo C, Drago F, Caraci F. 'Role of Omega-3 Fatty Acids in the Treatment of Depressive Disorders: A Comprehensive Meta-Analysis of Randomized Clinical Trials'. *Public Library of Science*, 2014, Volume 9(5): e96905.

Hankey GJ, Ford AH, Yi Q, Eikelboom JW, Lees KR, Chen C, Xavier D, Navarro JC, Ranawaka UK, Uddin W, Ricci S, Gommans J, Schmidt R, Almeida OP, van Bockxmeer FM; VITATOPS Trial Study Group. 'Effect of B vitamins and lowering homocysteine on cognitive impairment in patients with previous stroke or transient ischemic attack: a prespecified secondary analysis of a randomized, placebo-controlled trial and meta-analysis'. *Stroke,* 2013, Volume 44(8):2232-9.

Fava M, Alpert J, Nierenberg AA, Mischoulon D, Otto MW, Zajecka J, Murck H, Rosenbaum JF. 'A Double-blind, randomized trial of St John's wort, fluoxetine, and placebo in major depressive disorder.' *Journal of Clinical Psychopharmacology*, 2005, Volume 25(5):441-7.

Herrschaft H, Nacu A, Likhachev S, Sholomov I, Hoerr R, Schlaefke S Ginkgo biloba extract EGb 761® in dementia with neuropsychiatric features: A randomised, placebo-controlled trial to confirm the efficacy and safety of a daily dose of 240 mg'. *Journal of Psychiatric Research*, 2012, Volume 46(6):716-723

Hirayama S, Terasawa K, Rabeler R, Hirayama T, Inoue T, Tatsumi Y, Purpura M, Jäger R. 'The effect of phosphatidylserine administration on memory and symptoms of attention-deficit hyperactivity disorder: a randomised, double-blind, placebo-controlled clinical trial.' *Journal of Human Nutrition and Dietetics*, 2014, Volume 27, Supplement 2:284-91.

Kidd PM 'Alzheimer's Disease, Amnestic Mild Cognitive Impairment, and Age-Associated Memory Impairment: Current Understanding and Progress Toward Integrative Prevention'. *Alternative Medicine Review*, 2009, Volume 13, issue 2: 85-115.

Kirsch I, Deacon BJ, Huedo-Medina TB, Scoboria A, Moore TJ, Johnson BT, 'Initial Severity and Antidepressant Benefits: A Meta-Analysis of Data Submitted to the Food and Drug Administration'. *Public Library of Science Medicine*, 2008, Volume 5(2): e45.

Königs A, Kiliaan AJ, 'Critical appraisal of omega-3 fatty acids in attention-deficit/hyperactivity disorder treatment'. *Neuropsychiatric disease and treatment*, 2016, Volume 12: 1869–1882.

Lopresti AL, Hood SD, Drummond PD. 'A review of lifestyle factors that contribute to important pathways associated with major depression: diet, sleep and exercise'. *Journal of Affective Disorders*, 2013, Volume 148(1):12-27.

Moré MI, Freitas U, Rutenberg D. 'Positive effects of soy lecithin-derived phosphatidylserine plus phosphatidic acid on memory, cognition, daily functioning, and mood in elderly patients with Alzheimer's disease and dementia.' *Advances in Therapy,* 2014, Volume 31(12):1247-62.

Patrick RP, Ames BN. 'Vitamin D and the omega-3 fatty acids control serotonin synthesis and action, part 2: relevance for ADHD, bipolar disorder, schizophrenia, and impulsive behaviour.' *FASEB Journal*, 2015, Volume 29(6):2207-22.

Santos C, Costa J, Santos J, Vaz-Carneiro A, Lunet N. 'Caffeine intake and dementia: systematic review and meta-analysis'. *Journal of Alzheimer's Disease*, 2010, Volume 20 Supplement 1:S187-204.

Scott TM, Rogers G, Weiner DE, Livingston K, Selhub J, Jacques PF, Rosenberg IH, Troen AM. 'B-Vitamin Therapy for Kidney Transplant Recipients Lowers Homocysteine and Improves Selective Cognitive Outcomes in the Randomized FAVORIT Ancillary Cognitive Trial'. *The Journal of Prevention of Alzheimer's Disease*, 2017, Volume 4(3):174-182.

Shen L, Ji HF. 'Vitamin D deficiency is associated with increased risk of Alzheimer's disease and dementia: evidence from meta-analysis.' *Nutrition Journal,* 2015, Volume 14:76.

Skarupski KA, Tangney C, Li H, Ouyang B, Evans DA, Morris MC. 'Longitudinal association of vitamin B-6, folate, and vitamin B-12 with depressive symptoms among older adults over time'. *American Journal of Clinical Nutrition*, 2010, Volume 92(2): 330–335.

Smith AD, Smith SM, de Jager CA, Whitbread P, Johnston C, Agacinski G, Oulhaj A, Bradley KM, Jacoby R, Refsum H. 'Homocysteine-Lowering by B Vitamins Slows the Rate of Accelerated Brain Atrophy in Mild Cognitive Impairment: A Randomized Controlled Trial'. *Public Library of Science One*, 2010, Volume 5(9): e12244.

Ventriglia M, Brewer GJ, Simonelli I, Mariani S, Siotto M, Bucossi S, Squitti R. 'Zinc in Alzheimer's Disease: A Meta-Analysis of Serum, Plasma, and Cerebrospinal Fluid Studies'. *Journal of Alzheimer's Disease*, 2015, Volume 46(1):75-87.

White DJ, Cox KHM, RPeters R, Pipingas A, Scholey AB. 'Effects of Four-Week Supplementation with a Multi-Vitamin/Mineral Preparation on Mood and Blood Biomarkers in Young Adults: A Randomised, Double-Blind, Placebo-Controlled Trial'. *Nutrients*, 2015, Volume 7(11): 9005–9017.

Wong SK, Chin KY, Ima-Nirwana S. 'Vitamin D and Depression: The Evidence from an Indirect Clue to Treatment Strategy'. *Current Drug Targets*, 2018, Volume 19(8):888-897.

Yoon S, Cho H, Kim J, Lee D, Kim GH, Hong YS, Moon S, Park S, Lee S, Lee S, Bae S, Simonson DC, Lyoo IK, 'Brain changes in overweight/obese and normal-weight adults with type 2 diabetes mellitus'. *Diabetologia*, 2017, Volume 60, Issue 7, pp 1207–1217.

Zheng Z, Wang J, Yi L, Yu H, Kong L, Cui W, Chen H, Wang C. 'Correlation between behavioural and psychological symptoms of Alzheimer type dementia and plasma homocysteine concentration'. *Biomed Research International*, 2014, Volume 2014:383494.

Digestion

Arjoon AV, Saylor CV, May M. 'In Vitro efficacy of antimicrobial extracts against the atypical ruminant pathogen Mycoplasma mycoides subsp. capri.' *BMC Complementary and Alternative Medicine*, 2012, Volume 12:169.

Attaluri A, Donahoe R, Valestin J, Brown K, Rao SS. 'Randomised clinical trial: dried plums (prunes) vs. psyllium for constipation.' *Alimentary Pharmacology and Therapeutics*, 2011 Volume 33(7):822-8.

Brown R, Sam CH, Green T, Wood S. Effect of GutsyGum(tm), A Novel Gum, on 'Subjective Ratings of Gastro Esophageal RefluxFollowing A Refluxogenic Meal.' *Journal of Dietary Supplements*, 2015, Volume 12(2):138-45.

de Oliveira Leite AM, Miguel MA, Peixoto RS, Rosado AS, Silva JT, Paschoalin VM. 'Microbiological, technological and therapeutic properties of kefir: a natural probiotic beverage.' *Brazilian Journal of Microbiology*, 2013, Volume 44(2):341-9.

Didari T, Mozaffari S, Nikfar S, Abdollahi M. 'Effectiveness of probiotics in irritable bowel syndrome: Updated systematic review with meta-analysis.' *World Journal of Gastroenterolgy,* 2015, Volume 21(10):3072-84.

Jarosz M, Taraszewska A. 'Risk factors for gastroesophageal reflux disease: the role of diet'. *Przeglad Gastroenterologiczny*, 2014, Volume 9(5):297-301.

Jones VA, McLaughlan P, Shorthouse M, Workman E, Hunter JO.'Food intolerance: a major factor in the pathogenesis of irritable bowel syndrome'. *Lancet*, 1982, Volume 2, Issue 8308: 1115-7.

Kubo A, Block G, Quesenberry CP, Buffler P, Corley DA, 'Dietary guideline adherence for gastroesophageal reflux disease'. *BMC Gastroenterology*, 2014, Volume 14: 144.

Lee EH, Park CW, Jung YJ. 'Anti-inflammatory and immune-modulating effect of Ulmus davidiana var. japonica Nakai extract on a macrophage cell line and immune cells in the mouse small intestine.' *Journal of Ethnopharmacology,* 2013, Volume 146(2):608-13.

Lee HS, Jang MS, Kim JH, Hong CP, Lee EJ, Jeun EJ, Kim C, Kim EK, Ahn KS, Yang BG, Ahn KS, Jang YP, Ahn KS, Kim YM, Jang MH. 'Ulmus davidiana var. japonica Nakai upregulates eosinophils and suppresses Th1 and Th17 cells in the small intestine.' *Public Library of Science*, 2013, Volume 8(10):e76716.

Nanda R, James R, Smith H, Dudley CR, Jewell DP. 'Food intolerance and the irritable bowel syndrome'. *Gut,* 1989, Volume 30, Issue 8: 1099-104.

Rosa DD, Dias MMS, Grześkowiak ŁM, Reis SA, Conceição LL, Peluzio MDCG. 'Milk kefir: nutritional, microbiological and health benefits.' *Nutrition Research Reviews*, 2017, Volume 30(1):82-96.

Sharifi-Rad M, Varoni EM2, Iriti M, Martorell M, Setzer WN, Del Mar Contreras M, Salehi B, Soltani-Nejad A, Rajabi S, Tajbakhsh M, Sharifi-Rad J. 'Carvacrol and human health: A comprehensive review.' *Phytotherapy Research*, May 2018 [Epub ahead of print].

Shepherd SJ, Gibson PR. 'Fructose malabsorption and symptoms of irritable bowel syndrome: guidelines for effective dietary management.' *Journal of the American Dietetic Association*, 2006, Volume106(10):1631-9.

Skin conditions

Adebamowo CA, Spiegelman D, Berkey CS, Danby FW, Rockett HH, Colditz GA, Willett WC, Holmes MD. 'Milk consumption and acne in adolescent girls.' *Dermatology Online Journal,* 2006, Volume 12(4):1.

Bamford JT, Ray S, Musekiwa A, van Gool C, Humphreys R, Ernst E. 'Oral evening primrose oil and borage oil for eczema.' *Cochrane Database of Systematic Reviews,* 2013, Volume (4):CD004416.

Burris J, Rietkerk W, Shikany JM, Woolf K. 'Differences in Dietary Glycemic Load and Hormones in New York City Adults with No and Moderate/Severe Acne.' *Journal of the Academy of Nutrition and Dietetics*, 2017, Volume 117(9):1375-1383.

Chan H, Chan G, Santos J, Dee K, Co JK. 'A randomized, double-blind, placebo-controlled trial to determine the efficacy and safety of lactoferrin with vitamin E and zinc as an oral therapy for mild to moderate acne vulgaris.' *International Journal of Dermatology*, 2017, Volume 56(6):686-690.

De Bastiani R, Gabrielli M, Lora L, Napoli L, Tosetti C, Pirrotta E, Ubaldi E, Bertolusso L, Zamparella M, De Polo M, Nebiacolombo C, Bortot M, Mancuso M, Bacchin P, Marsala V, Pinna R, Tursi A, Benedetto E, Cuffari A, Pati A, Di Caro S, Perenzin G, Sala R, Calzavara Pinton G, Gasbarrini A. 'Association between coeliac disease and psoriasis: Italian primary care multicentre study.' *Dermatology*, 2015, Volume 230(2):156-60.

El-Akawi Z, Abdel-Latif N and Abdul-Razzak K. 'Does the plasma level of vitamins A and E affect acne condition?' *Clinical and Experimental Dermatology*, 2006, Volume 31, Issue 3: 430-4.

Ismail NH, Manaf ZA, Azizan NZ. 'High glycemic load diet, milk and ice cream consumption are related to acne vulgaris in Malaysian young adults: a case control study.' *BMC Dermatology*, 2012, Volume 12:13.

Kim JE, Yoo SR, Jeong MG, Ko JY, Ro YS. 'Hair zinc levels and the efficacy of oral zinc supplementation in patients with atopic dermatitis.' *Acta Dermato Venereologica*, 2014, Volume 94(5):558-62.

Koch C, Dölle S, Metzger M, Rasche C, Jungclas H, Rühl R, Renz H, and Worm M. 'Docosahexaenoic acid (DHA) supplementation in atopic eczema: a randomized, double-blind, controlled trial'. *The British Journal of Dermatology*, 2008, Volume 158, Issue 4: 786-792.

Magnusson J, Kull I, Rosenlund H, Håkansson N, Wolk A, Melén E, Wickman M, Bergström A. 'Fish consumption in infancy and development of allergic disease up to age 12 y.' *American Journal of Clinical Nutrition*, 2013, Volume 97(6):1324-30.

Mahmood SN, Bowe WP. 'Diet and acne update: carbohydrates emerge as the main culprit.' *Journal of Drugs in Dermatology*, 2014, Volume 13(4):428-35.

Mansfield JA, Bergin SW, Cooper JR, Olsen CH. 'Comparative probiotic strain efficacy in the prevention of eczema in infants and children: a systematic review and meta-analysis.' *Military Medicine*, 2014, Volume 179(6):580-92.

Melnik B. 'Milk consumption: aggravating factor of acne and promoter of chronic diseases of Western societies.' *Journal of the German Society of Dermatology*, 2009, Volume 7(4):364-70.

Merola JF, Han J, Li T, Qureshi AA. 'No association between vitamin D intake and incident psoriasis among US women.' *Archives of Dermatological Research*, 2014, Volume 306(3):305-7.

Nosrati A, Afifi L, Danesh MJ, Lee K, Yan D, Beroukhim K, Ahn R, Liao W. 'Dietary modifications in atopic dermatitis: patient-reported outcomes.' *The Journal of Dermatological Treatment*, 2017 Volume 28(6):523-538.

Notay M, Foolad N, Vaughn AR, Sivamani RK. 'Probiotics, Prebiotics, and Synbiotics for the Treatment and Prevention of Adult Dermatological Diseases.' *American Journal of Clinical Dermatology*, 2017, Volume 18(6):721-732.

Ozuguz P, Dogruk Kacar S, Ekiz O, Takci Z, Balta I, Kalkan G. 'Evaluation of serum vitamins A and E and zinc levels according to the severity of acne vulgaris.' *Cutaneous and Ocular Toxicology*, 2014, Volume 33(2):99-102.

Schlichte MJ, Vandersall A, Katta R. 'Diet and eczema: a review of dietary supplements for the treatment of atopic dermatitis.' *Dermatology Practical and Conceptual,* 2016, Volume 6(3):23-9.

Smith RN, Mann NJ, Braue A, Mikelainen H. and Varigos GA 'The effect of a high-protein, low glycemic–load diet versus a conventional, high glycemic–load diet on biochemical parameters associated with acne vulgaris: A randomized, investigator-masked, controlled trial'. *Journal of the American Academy of Dermatology*, 2007, Volume 57, Issue 2: 247-256.

Soleymani T, Hung T, Soung J. 'The role of vitamin D in psoriasis: a review.' *International Journal of Dermatology*, 2015, Volume 54(4):383-92.

Spencer EH, Ferdowsian HR, Barnard ND, 'Diet and acne: a review of the evidence.' *International Journal of Dermatology*, 2009, Volume 48(4):339-347.

Tanaka T, Kouda K, Kotani M, Takeuchi A, Tabei T, Masamoto Y, Nakamura H, Takigawa M, Suemura M, Takeuchi H. and Kouda M. 'Vegetarian diet ameliorates symptoms of atopic dermatitis through reduction of the number of peripheral eosinophils and of PGE2 synthesis by monocytes'. *Journal of Physiological Anthropology and Applied Human Science*, 2001, Volume 20, Issue 6: 353-61.

Uehara M, Sugiura H, Sakurai K. 'A trial of oolong tea in the management of recalcitrant atopic dermatitis'. *Archives of Dermatology*, 2001, Volume 137, Issue 1: 42-3.

Websites

Arthritis and osteoporosis

www.arthritiscare.org.uk
A website covering all types of arthritis, providing information on what arthritis is and how to live with it, and listing other publications and resources. It also provides information on national and local events and support, with an arthritis care helpline.

www.arthritisresearchuk.org
A website covering all types of arthritis as well as other bone, joint and muscle related conditions such as osteoporosis, back pain, gout and fibromyalgia. There are video links so you can watch and listen to information on each condition rather than read information on the website.

www.nos.org.uk
This is the website for the National Osteoporosis Society. It offers a range of information including useful information leaflets on other medical conditions and treatments that may contribute to osteoporosis, and excellent leaflets on exercise and what to eat for good bone health.

www.ukgoutsociety.org
A website providing information on and help for gout sufferers.

Diabetes

https://www.diabetes.co.uk
A website offering a wealth of information on all types of diabetes, plus a blood sugar converter (mg/dl to mmol/l), tools such as body mass index (BMI) calculators and access to a free lifestyle site where you can monitor your blood glucose, blood pressure, weight and BMI and use a food diary and carb counter to help adjust your diet.

www.diabetes.org.uk
This website features a host of information and support tools including recipes, information on carbohydrate counting and a brilliant shopping and menu planning tool which provides information about each type of food and its benefits and drawbacks for diabetes.

Heart disease and related conditions

www.bhf.org.uk
An extensive website providing a wide variety of information, recipes and video clips as well as links to other useful, related websites, and tools such as a BMI calculator.

www.bpassoc.org.uk
A website providing written and video/audio information on blood pressure – what it is, how to measure it, and how to keep it within a healthy range.

Digestion

https://www.kcl.ac.uk/lsm/Schools/life-course-sciences/ departments/nutritional-sciences/projects/fodmaps/faq.aspx
Researchers at Kings College, London adapted the original FODMAP diet from Australia for UK use. Visit this web link for more information on the FODMAP diet.

Mental health conditions

www.fabresearch.org
A great website for information, fact sheets and research on conditions where behaviour, learning and mood are linked with food and nutrition, such as attention deficit hyperactivity disorder, dyslexia, dyspraxia, depression and ageing and mental health.

http://www.foodforthebrain.org
Food for the Brain are a charitable foundation working to inform organisations and empower individuals to change their diet and lifestyle and take greater control of their own mental health. They have an online Cognitive Function test you can do which gives you immediate feedback on your cognitive function, and some pointers on diet relating to the information you have input about your diet and lifestyle. If you score low in the Cognitive Function test, it may be worth getting your homocysteine levels checked by your GP.

www.mentalhealth.org.uk
This website offers a wide range of information on mental health conditions, as well as podcasts for general wellbeing and the latest news and research on mental health.

General health information

www.medicinenet.com

https://www.netdoctor.co.uk

http://www.nhs.co.uk

https://www.bupa.co.uk